# How to Grow a Garden of

# MEDICINAL HEALING PLANTS AND HERBS

## Learn How to Plant, Grow, Harvest & Store all Natural Botanicals Indoors & Outdoor

By

## CHRISTOPHER SPICER

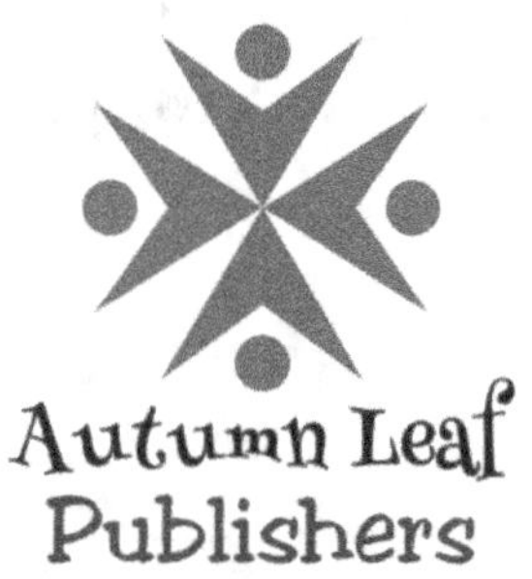


Design & Illustration by Robin Wright

First Edition

# CONTENTS

# Growing and Using Medicinal Herbs and Plants: Introduction

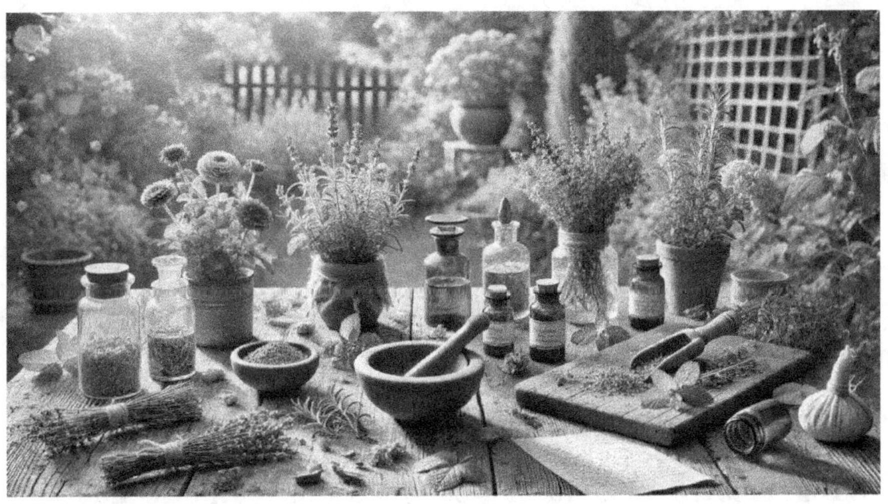

For thousands of years, the world relied on herbal medicine before the invention of modern medicine. Most common diseases were adequately treated or managed by using herbs that are readily available in our gardens. It was not until about 200 years ago that the world started using what we now call conventional medicine. However, shifting from herbal to conventional medicine has left some gaps that are yet to be filled. Modern medicine might be the best option for treating most ailments. Still, it fails at answering critical questions about some common diseases. Thankfully, we can always use traditional herbs to treat, manage, or prevent most of the ailments that conventional medicine is unable to treat.

Growing up, I encountered herbs more than an average kid. My grandmother was an herbal doctor, running an unregistered herbal clinic from her farm. Whenever we visited her, we would meet patients of all sorts coming in and asking questions about various herbs. Her garden was decorated with many types of plants, some of which I have not seen since she passed away. Her beautiful garden and treatment methods sparked my interest in herbal treatments. Having been a science fanatic at school, I aimed to disapprove of her treatment methods. I wanted to research more about the concoctions she was handling and let her know that she was just serving her customers with some bitter soup.

Unfortunately, my grandmother died while I was in high school. She had lived for about 80 years, and she was still full of vitality at the time of her death. When I went to college, I chose to focus on botanical research. I wanted to understand more about herbs and their authenticity as medical products. For the past two and a half decades, I have been researching, studying, and testing different types of herbs as medicine. Decades of research down the line, I have come to appreciate the medicinal value of most herbs, some of which we encounter every day.

Through research, I have come to appreciate the fact that most herbal treatments are more helpful than conventional medicine. They do not have side effects and are cheaper compared to herbal medicine. Looking back, now I understand why my grandmother remained healthy to the age of 80. Today, I cannot name a single woman as strong as she was past the age of 60. In a nutshell, herbal medicine works and is much better in sustaining life than pharmaceutical medicine.

In this book, we are going to walk through a journey of discovering herbal medicine. If you have an interest in herbalism, gardening, and backyard herbal farming, this is your book. I have divided this book into 4 main sections.

The first section of the book gives you an introduction to herbalism. If you are new to the world of herbal treatments, I will help you figure out what herbal medicine means and why it is important. We will look at a brief history of herbal medicine, what herbal medicine truly means, the benefits of herbal treatments, and the disadvantages.

In the second section of the book, we focus on growing herbal plants. Although many people are interested in using herbal medicines, a few can access the needed herbs. The book will help you learn how to plant herbs at home and determine the right herbs to plant. We will look at the best herbal plants to grow based on your climate zone. We will carry out a full review of the available climate zones in North America and how they may affect specific types of plants.

In the third section of the book, we will look at the best ways to use herbal plants. All the plants we have discussed how to grow and harvest in section two above will be utilized in treating various ailments. We will look at recipes for preparing treatments from these herbs. We will also look at the dosage of the herbs, the application process, and the best practices when using such herbal remedies.

In the last section, we will focus on precautions to be taken when applying for herbal medicine. Just like conventional drugs, some herbal medicine might have side effects. This book gives you a detailed outlook on the medicinal plants that you may use without fear. We also look at the plants that we must take precautions when using. Finally, we review the risks involved in using particular medicine for specific individuals.

If you are enthusiastic about herbal medicine, this book is for you. The book caters to all those who have an interest in maintaining a healthy lifestyle, treating chronic conditions, and those who only want to learn more about herbs. The book also serves those who are interested in backyard horticulture and herb farming. Welcome aboard, and let us ride this train together.

# Chapter 1: Understanding Horticulture and Herbalism

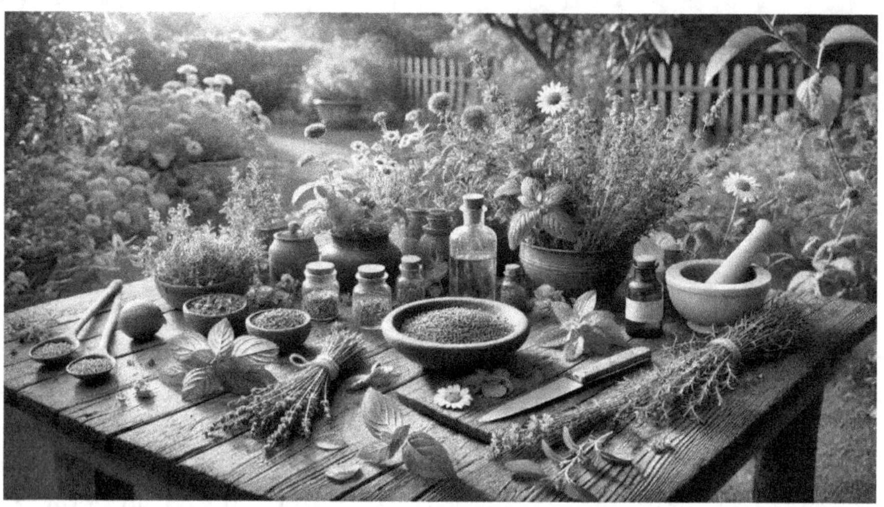

What is herbal medicine?

Herbal medicine refers to the study and application of medicinal plants in treating ailments and maintaining a healthy lifestyle. Herbal medicine has its roots in human history, with specific plants having preferred in particular cultures. The discovery of the medicinal value of specific plants has to be traced down to certain cultures in history. However, the application of herbal medicine is no longer made blindly. Traditionally, herbs were applied on a wait and see basis. In other words, herbs were used to determine if they could treat a specific condition. If an herb turned out to be a treatment for a particular ailment, it was adopted.

Today, herbal medicine goes beyond the scope of observation. Treatments are now considered through the scientific research process. Before an herb is termed as being of medicinal value, laboratory tests have to be done, and the accurate usage of the plant determined.

In recent years, many researchers have been digging out information regarding some of the known herbal plants. Before the 21st century, most people had assumed that herbal medicine does not have value in the modern world. However, recent studies are now showing that herbs are potent with medicinal compounds that can treat most ailments.

While most herbs have active medicinal compounds, it is not ideal to attempt to isolate the compounds from the plant. In my years of research, I have noticed that most active compounds lose their potency when separated from the main plant. This is the reason why herbal medicine is consumed naturally. In most cases, herbal medicine has to be consumed in its natural form. For example, salicylic acid is a compound found in meadowsweet. This compound is used in making aspirin - a pharmaceutical drug. One of the major side effects of taking aspirin is that it can lead to stomach bleeding. However, taking meadowsweet does not have any side effects but offers the same medicinal value as aspirin. In other words, herbal medicine works the best and has fewer side effects as compared to conventional medicine. In herbal treatments, therapeutic compounds are mostly consumed in the natural state of the plant to reduce associated side effects.

The primary aim of using herbal medicine is not to treat a specific ailment but is to return the body to its natural state. Herbal medicine works best when used to maintain a healthy lifestyle and to control diseases. However, many herbs are used to treat specific conditions, as we will see later on.

All herbal plants have potent medicinal compounds that must be taken cautiously. Most pharmaceutical medications are made based on these naturally occurring compounds. It is, therefore, necessary to take herbal medicine with caution.

Herbal medicines are mistakenly thought to be 100% safe just because they are natural. This is a misconception that does not have any scientific backing. There are plenty of natural herbs that are poisonous and harmful to humans. Some medicinal plants can produce adverse effects such as allergic reactions, vomiting, nausea, and diarrhea, among others. Just like the case with conventional medicine, herbal drugs should be taken cautiously. You should only take the right dosage at the right time. With that said, most herbal medications do not have side effects.

As we will see later, using herbal medicine with pharmaceutical drugs can lead to adverse effects. Herbal drugs should be used independently and should never be combined with conventional medications. However, if you are already using herbal medicine and have to use pharmaceutical drugs, you should talk to your doctor. The other factors you have to consider while using your herbal drugs include pregnancy, heart diseases, and diabetes, among others. As we move on, we will have a detailed look at various medicinal plants and how they can help maintain a healthy body.

# THE BENEFITS OF NATURAL REMEDIES VS. MAINSTREAM PHARMACEUTICALS

There are always questions as to whether herbal medicine is a better option as compared to pharmaceutical drugs. The question of whether to go herbal or pharmaceutical cannot be answered conclusively. However, you should never have to choose between the two. Each of the options has its benefits and disadvantages. With that being said, herbal drugs are preferred by those who champion for natural ways of treatment. They have many benefits and fewer side effects as compared to conventional medicines. Some of the benefits of herbal drugs as compared to conventional medications include:

Herbal drugs are not limited to treating diseases. If you choose to make herbs part of your life, you can use them on a daily basis. Some herbs can be used to maintain a naturally healthy body without necessarily treating diseases. For instance, garlic is an herbal medicine, but it is also used as a cooking spice. The spice helps improve blood flow and reduce the possibility of heart disease. The same cannot be said about pharmaceutical medicine. Most conventional drugs are designed to treat a condition once it occurs. They cannot be used as a part of your lifestyle to control the occurrence of diseases.

## HERBAL DRUGS ARE NATURAL AND HAVE FEWER SIDE EFFECTS.

The other benefit of herbal drugs is that they have fewer side effects. The main reason for having fewer effects is that herbal medicines are natural. As we have already seen, herbal drugs are used in their natural form. The medicinal compounds used in a natural way do not have side effects as the case where they are extracted. We have looked at the instance of aspirin, where salicylic acid can cause bleeding. However, if the same acid is consumed in natural foods, it does not have the same effects.

## HERBAL DRUGS ARE MUCH CHEAPER AND READILY AVAILABLE.

The other benefit of herbal drugs is that they are cheap and readily available. You can plant all types of herbs at home and use them to take care of your family. The same cannot be said about pharmaceutical drugs. In most cases, pharmaceutical drugs need substantial investment in terms of money. Most drugs are developed by pharmaceutical companies that are out to make hefty profits. However, herbal medications can be obtained at a lower price. Even if you do not have a farm to plant most of the herbs, you can easily purchase them from local grocery stores or farmer's markets.

## HERBAL DRUGS ARE ACCESSIBLE.

The other benefit of herbal drugs over pharmaceutical options is accessibility. Pharmaceutical drugs are only available in developed regions with modern medical facilities. If you happen to reside in a locality with limited access to modern medical facilities, you will have a hard time accessing pharmaceutical drugs. However, herbal medicine can be grown and nurtured at home. Even if you live in the most remote part of the world, you will have access to natural remedies.

## HERBAL MEDICINE IS APPLICABLE IN MANY FORMS.

The other benefit of herbal medicine is the diverse procedure of application. While pharmaceutical drugs come in many forms, they cannot be compared to herbal medications. With herbaceous plants, the same drug can be used to prepare herbal tea, salves, oils, or can be consumed directly. If you are not comfortable with swallowing pills, you can easily choose to brew tea with your herbs. In other words, herbs can be consumed either as food, via topical applications, or as a drug through direct ingestion. This makes it possible to apply herbal medicines to all people, even children.

The other benefit of herbal medicine is that it is preventive. Most people who use herbs use them for prevention and management rather than treatment. I mentioned that my grandmother lived to the age of 80. Today, few people can barely live past the age of 60. The main reason why those who rely on traditional medicine live longer is that the drugs are preventive. These drugs help your body maintain a natural balance and help detoxify the body of any harmful substance. Most herbal remedies are not focused on treating an already existing condition but instead stopping the condition before it happens. This approach to human health is much better than treating disease. Prevention helps stop the possibility of the disease occurring, and it keeps a person healthy for long. With pharmaceutical medicine, there are no prescriptions for maintaining a healthy body. Pharmaceutical drugs are usually focused on treating a specific condition at the time it occurs. This approach can lead to a myriad of health complications and often leads to a shortened lifespan.

# Glossary of Terms for Horticulture, Backyard Agriculture, and Herbal Medicine

**Acid Soil**: Refers to a soil that has a pH below 7. In other words, the soil has more acidic compounds than basic compounds.

**Acuminate**: Gradually tapering to an elongated point.

**Agamic**: This refers to a situation where you reproduce a plant without using seeds. For instance, you can cut the stem of an already growing plant and transfer it to a different region.

**Air Layering**: This refers to a type of vegetation propagation approach, where a specially treated part of a branch is enclosed until roots emerge. Once the roots are developed, the plant is detached from the main branch and planted.

**Alkaline Soil**: Refers to soil with a pH above 7. It is the opposite of acidic soil in that the soil has more basic compounds.

**Alternate**: This term is used to refer to a pattern of leaves on the stem, where the leaves are arranged at different heights.

**Amplexicaul:** This refers to a situation where the base of the leaf covers the stem.

**Anemophilous**: This refers to wind-pollinated plants.

**Balled and Bur lapped**: This term is used to describe a plant that is ready for transplanting with burlap wrapped soil around its base.

**Bare Root**: This term describes a plant that is ready for transplanting without protective soil covering its roots.

**Bearded**: Refers to a plant that is furnished with long hairs.

**Biennial**: The term is used to describe a plant that lives for two years or developing seasons. It produces leaves in the first season and flowers and seeds in the second season.

**Candle**: This refers to the young new bud-like shoot that sends out young needles on the conifer.

**Cane**: A long, sweet, supple stem of grass-like vegetation.

**Capitate**: This refers to a group of plants or fruits that collect into a cluster.

**Capsulate**: This refers to a dry dehiscent fruit that opens up on ripening and disperses its seeds. Such plants naturally grow since the seeds are planted on the ground once the fruits mature.

**Capsule**: This refers to dry fruit containing seeds. The term can also be used to refer to a medicinal tablet having more than one cover.

**Carpel**: This refers to the part of a flower that produces seeds.

**Dioecious**: This refers to plants that bear male flowers on one plant and female flowers on a different plant.

**Direct Seeding**: This refers to a situation where the seeds are directly planted into the garden instead of preparing a nursery first.

**Disbud**: This refers to removing buds from flowers to encourage them to produce more flowers.

**Dissected**: This term refers to dividing land or a garden into many small segments. This approach works the best with backyard herbal farming due to the large variety of herbs to be planted.

**Divaricate**: This refers to a situation where a branch goes out in a totally different direction from the other branches.

**Drupe**: This refers to fruit with a fleshy part with and a single hard seed in the middle. A good example would be an avocado.

**Dwarf**: This refers to a shrub that is short in height, usually less than 3 feet.

**Emarginate**: A plant with a shallow notch at the apex.

**Espalier**: Refers to the process of training a plant to grow flat along with a structure in a decorative manner. This approach is usually used with climbing plants.

**Evergreen**: This refers to a plant that retains its leaves throughout the year. It does not change shades or dry leaves even when seasons change.

**Exfoliate**: This term is used to refer to a fruit or stem that loses the outer cover naturally.

**Family**: The term family refers to a group of plants that share the same physical features and compounds.

**Fastigiate**: Refers to a plant with branches that close together.

**Fertile**: Refers to a plant that can produce fruits and seeds. A plant that is referred to as being fertile can produce young ones in the long run.

**Fertilizer**: A mix used to supply nutrients to plants and enhance their growth. There are different types of fertilizer, and they serve different purposes.

**Hardy**: This term refers to plants that can withstand harsh temperatures, especially cold winters.

**Hastate**: This refers to plants with a broad but pointed apex.

**Herbaceous**: This refers to an herb that completely dies down after flowering. It is a seasonal flower that flourishes during the spring and summer.

**Herbaceous**: This refers to a plant that lacks a woody structure.

**Hermaphrodite**: This refers to female and male flowers in the same inflorescence.

**Heterophyllies**: A type of plant that produces different kinds of leaves and flowers.

**Indehiscent**: A plant that does not open up the seeds when the fruit is ripe. In other words, the seeds are contained within the shell even if the fruit is ripe.

**Inflorescence**: The term refers to flowers and the flower stalk when grouped together.

**Infructescence**: This refers to fruits formed from the inflorescence.

**Lace Bug**: Insects with broad, lacy wings that suck sap from flowers.

**Amoebicidal**: This refers to herbs that are used to treat conditions caused by amoeba such as amoebic dysentery.

**Analgesic or Anodynes**: These are herbs that are used to reduce or eliminate pain-causing illness. For instance, chamomile, lavender, cloves, and other anti-inflammatory herbs can reduce inflammation of any kind and consequently soothe the pain.

**Anaphrodisiac**: These are herbs that are used to delay sexual desire, especially in men. They can be used to prolong the duration of a man during a sexual encounter.

**Anesthetics**: Refer to herbs that can induce numbness to a specific part of the body. Some of the herbs in this category include Ashok and Gudmar. Such herbs are used to reduce pain or make an individual numb during a painful procedure such as childbirth or circumcision.

**Anthelmintic**: This term is used to refer to anti-parasitic herbs. Such herbs are used to destroy worms, fungus, and other parasites that may want to live on your body. Some examples of anti-parasitic herbs include wormwood, goldenseal, and cayenne pepper.

**Anodyne**: These are pain-relieving herbs and can be used to reduce all types of pain, including joint, muscle, and wound pains. Examples of such herbs include Ashok, cedar, and ginger.

**Antacid**: These are herbs that are used to neutralize excess stomach acids. Some examples of antacid herbs include marshmallow root, meadowsweet herb, and hops flowers.

**Ant bilious**: These are herbs that are used to combat nausea, stomach ache, and bilious symptoms caused by secretion of excess bile.

**Antibiotic**: These are herbs that help prevent the growth of bacteria. Some examples of antibiotic herbs include turmeric and Echinacea.

**Antidepressant:** This term refers to herbs that offer a mentally soothing effect to counter mental health problems such as depression.

**Antidiabetic**: Refers to herbs that help the body utilize insulin more effectively. Such herbs are used to treat diabetes and insulin imbalance related conditions. Some examples of such herbs include Amalaka, blackberry, and gummer.

**Antidiarrheal**: This refers to drugs that stop diarrhea. Some examples of anti-diarrhea herbs include comfrey, gentian, red raspberry, and yellow dock, among others.

**Antiemetic**: These are herbs that prevent nausea and vomiting. Some examples of antiemetic herbs include cloves, coriander, ginger, and raspberry.

**Antiepileptic**: This refers to herbs that can combat epileptic fits or seizures.

**Anti-hemorrhagic**: This refers to drugs that can prevent or alleviate hemorrhaging.

**Anti-inflammatory:** This refers to herbs that reduce inflammation. Most medical conditions are caused by inflammation and can be treated with anti-inflammatory herbs.

**Anti-lithic:** This refers to herbs that prevent the formation of kidney stones and bladder stones.

**Anti-periodic**: This refers to herbs that prevent the periodic occurrence of diseases such as malaria. Some examples of anti-periodic herbs include barberry and Kuta.

**Antiphlogistic**: This refers to herbs that counter inflammation. They are also known as anti-inflammatories per the description above.

**Antipyretic:** These are herbs that reduce fever by destroying fever toxins. Such herbs induce perspiration and increase the loss of heat. Some examples of antipyretic herbs include Amalaka, black pepper, Brihati, and Nir gundi.

**Antirheumatic:** This refers to herbs that can reduce, manage, or cure rheumatism.

**Antiscorbutic**: This refers to herbs that are effective in treating, preventing, or controlling scurvy.

**Antiseptic:** This refers to herbs that prevent the development of microorganisms. Antiseptic compounds do not necessarily destroy microorganisms but rather stop their spread by creating an environment that does not allow the organisms to grow. Some examples of antiseptic herbs include aloe vera, Gohr, Gudmar, and turmeric, among others.

**Antispasmodic**: This refers to herbs that can reduce involuntary muscle spasms. Some examples of antispasmodic herbs include chamomile, basil, guggul, licorice, sage, and peppermint.

**Ant syphilitic**: This refers to herbs that are used to cure syphilis or control its spread. They are also known as antiluetics. Some examples of these herbs include cedar, black pepper, and guggul.

**Antitussive:** These are herbs that are used to prevent cough.

**Balsamic**: Balsamic refers to herbs that are used to soothe inflammation. Some examples include clary, sage, and avocado.

**Cell Proliferation:** This term is used to refer to herbs that boost immunity and restore an immune system that has been weakened by diseases.

**Cordials**: This term is used to refer to herbs that combine the properties of cardiac stimulating and stomach warming drugs. Some of the herbs that fall under this category include chamomile, rosemary, yarrow, lemongrass, and borage.

**Demulcents:** This refers to herbs that have mucilaginous properties. They are soothing and protective of internal tissues that are irritated and inflamed. Examples of such herbs include blue cohosh, comfrey root, mullein, and chickweed.

**Hypnotics**: This refers to herbs that are powerful nerve relaxants. Such herbs provide a relaxing effect to help people sleep well. Some examples of such herbs include mistletoe, valerian, and passionflower.

**Nephritis**: This refers to herbs that can protect, treat, or manage kidney conditions. Some of these plants include cayenne, cornsilk, and uva ursin.

**Nutritive**: This refers to herbs that nourish the body. Such herbs help in detoxifying the blood to enhance healthy functions. Some nutritious herbs include comfrey, mullein, slippery elm, sage, and sweet basil.

**Orexigenic**: This refers to herbs that stimulate the appetite. Most of these herbs are more potent than pharmaceutical drugs.

**Refrigerants**: This term is used to refer to herbs that relieve thirst with cooling properties. Some herbs under this category include chickweed, cleavers, elderflowers, and strawberries.

**Tonics**: This refers to herbs that stimulate, strengthen, and energize the body. Some of the herbs under this category include chicory, dandelions, thyme, and yarrow.

**Vermifuge:** This refers to herbs used to expel worms. They include aloe, blue cohosh, hyssop, and mandrake.

## WHAT PLANTS/HERBS ARE USEFUL FOR WHAT REMEDIES?

We are going to look at herbs in more detail as we move forward. For now, I just want us to look at a few of the common herbs and what they treat. There are thousands of herbs that can treat and manage various conditions. However, we will not be able to review all the herbs out there. For the purpose of this book, we will stick to the most potent herbs that can also be planted in our gardens. Some of the top-rated herbal remedies include:

**Chamomile**: Chamomile is a flower that is considered a cure-all by herbalists. This flower is an anxiolytic and sedative herb that helps in relaxation and curing mental conditions. It is used in European nations for healing wounds and reducing inflammation or swelling. Chamomile can be taken as a tea or applied as a compress. Although it is not approved as a drug, it is considered safe by the FDA. In other words, you will not get a chamomile prescription from conventional medical facilities. Still, you can prepare chamomile tea at home and help treat some of the conditions above.

**Echinacea**: Echinacea stalks or leaves can be used to treat common colds, flu, and infections. Several published studies have shown that this herb has healing properties when it comes to colds and flu. Some studies have revealed that long term use of the herb can help boost the overall body immune.

**Feverfew**: Feverfew is a medicinal herb that is used to treat fevers. It is commonly used in the US and Europe to prevent migraines and treat arthritis. The drug can be prepared to stop migraines at home. It may have some side effects such as mouth ulcers and digestive irritation. However, these effects do not occur in all people. If you start taking routine feverfew to control migraines, you may experience the headache return upon suddenly stopping the dosage. This drug should not be used with anticoagulants.

**Garlic**: Garlic is a spice that is mostly used in cooking. Its roots and cloves are known to have medicinal benefits. The spice is used to lower cholesterol level in the blood. It has an antimicrobial effect and, as a result, can act as an antiseptic. Reports from several studies have shown that garlic can reduce LDL cholesterol. This means that the spice can be used to lower the risk of heart diseases. Currently, there are studies underway to determine the role of garlic in controlling cancer. Although the FDA considers garlic safe, it does not recommend garlic as a drug. Garlic is safe for cooking and consumption.

**Ginger**: Ginger is another spice, whose roots are used to spice up various foods. This herb is known to have multiple health benefits, including reducing nausea and motion sickness. Several researchers have proved that ginger can reduce nausea caused by pregnancy or chemotherapy. The herb is also being investigated to determine the possibility of being used in surgery and nausea caused by motion. The herb can have some side effects such as bloating and excess gas.

**Gingko:** Gingko is a type of herb whose leaves can be used to treat asthma. The herb has also been found to be effective in the treatment and management of bronchitis, fatigue, and tinnitus. This herb is also used by old people to improve memory and treat dementia. Since dementia is a progressive disease, the herb should be made part of a daily lifestyle to reduce the chances of poor memory in the future. However, this herb might be toxic if the seeds are consumed. Only the leaves of the herb should be consumed in recommended dosages.

**Ginseng:** The other herb that is known and accepted as medicine is the ginseng root. This herb is used as a tonic and aphrodisiac. If you want to use ginseng to treat any condition, I recommend growing this plant. There are significant variations in the ginseng sold on the market. Although it is considered safe by the FDA, it should not be used with warfarin, heparin, and non-steroidal inflammatory (NSAID) medicines.

**Goldenseal**: Goldenseal is an herb that is used to treat common conditions. Its roots and rhizomes are used to treat diarrhea and skin irritation. It is also an antiseptic, which means that it can be used to treat the skin. Although several types of research are pointing toward its ability to treat colds, the facts are still scanty. Goldenseal contains berberine- an alkaloid substance that has been part of Chinese traditional medicine for long. Such substances and other compounds help this herb treat diarrhea and other stomach conditions. However, if this herb is taken in excess, it can be poisonous.

**Milk Thistle**: Milk thistle is a common treatment for liver conditions and high cholesterol. For this herb, the fruits contain the medicinal compounds. This herb has been used for many years to treat several conditions, primarily liver conditions.

**Saw Palmetto**: Saw palmetto is one of the most effective herbs. Its fruit is used to treat prostatic hypertrophy. Recent studies indicate that although it works well for treating this condition, it may have side effects such as stomach upsets in some people.

**Valerian**: The other herb that is commonly used as a medicine is valerian. It is used to manage conditions such as sleeplessness and to reduce anxiety. Research shows that valerian may help those who suffer from insomnia and stress-induced sleeplessness. In the US, valerian is mainly used as a flavoring root in beer and other foods. Although there are no documented side effects of this herb, talk to your doctor before using it.

# CHAPTER 2: GROWING THE HERBAL GARDEN

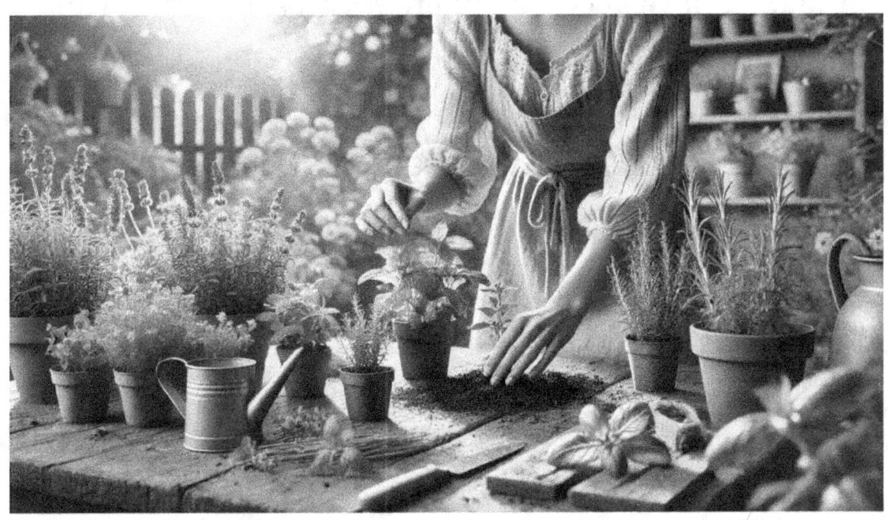

Now that we have looked at what herbal medicine entails, we are going to look at the technicalities involved in planting and maintaining an herbal garden. Since most of the herbs used as medicine are scarce, it is better to plant yours. Thankfully, most of the herbs can be matured at home, either indoors or outdoors. Even if you lack sufficient outdoor space, you can still grow some indoor herbs that are very helpful.

When planning your herb garden, you should start by selecting the herbs to plant. Although there are thousands of herbs you may plant, settle on a few. In our garden, we have about 30 different types of herbs. While 30 herbs may seem a few, they can treat almost all conditions you come across. For the purpose of this book, we will stick to plating about 25 types of herbs. I will help you select the best herbs that will treat most of the conditions. After selecting the herbs that you wish to plant, start designing your garden.

When selecting the plants to establish in your garden, it is important to consider their growth habits. If some plants mature faster than others, you will have to group those that mature slowly in one section and those that mature faster in a different section. You also have to consider the heights of the herbs and flowering habits. As much as herbal gardens are intended to offer herbs for medicinal value, the garden should also be decorative. This is very important, especially for those with a small backyard. If you lack the backyard space, we will look at other ways you can manage your garden. Here are some steps you can follow to design your garden and categorize your plants.

## CONSIDER COMPLEMENTARY COLORES AND CONTRASTING TEXTURES

Gardens are all about plant colors and flower types. It is important to pick plants that offer similar colors or contrasting leaf textures. For instance, you may keep your green section with green lavender flowers and spice them up with contrasting leaf textures such as the monarda.

However, since some of the green herbs might mature faster than others, you will need to do proper garden maintenance. For instance, if your green section combines lavender flowers with monarda, you have to deadhead the monarda to keep it in bloom longer. You can also use cilantro, which will help your garden flourish by self-seeding. However, you should note that the number of plants you include in your green section depends on the size of the garden. If your herb is small, you can use between 1 and 2 types of greens. For those with extensive

gardens, you may include as many green herbs in this
section as you wish.

## Introduce Colour and Flowers

After choosing your green and contrasting colors, settle on
colored flowers. Colored flowers will make the garden
beautiful. If the garden is in your front yard, you will
have to pay more attention to colored flowers. In this bed
include orange, yellow, blue, and purple flowers. In
general, any bright colored flower can fall under this
category. For instance, you could bring in borage- which
has electric blue flowers. Although self-seeding might
prove a problem, regular maintenance of the garden will
see it retain your intended look. You may choose to use
nasturtiums and chives on the edges. The other herbs you
may include in your colored flowers section include
parsley and calendula. These flowers will offer diversity
in colors and grow to almost similar heights.

After separating two beds of pure greens and colors, you can try playing around with several colors. If you have vast spaces in the backyard, you may try mixing up the colors and greens. However, the pattern of planting will play a role in this case. A mix-matched garden is easy to plant but may not look as good as you desire. In this section, you may want to include herbs that are contrasting in texture, foliage, and color. Purple sage is one of the herbs that looks great at all times of the year. You could make such an outstanding flower the center of the entire bed. You may also try to combine with some lavender just to bring in the spiky needle-like foliage. With a diverse bed, the aim is to try and combine different foliage, colors, textures, and much more. If you find a pattern that works, go for it and try to make your garden as beautiful as possible. However, consider the seasons and seeding of each herb you plant in this section.

When planning a garden, the focus should be at the center. You could divide your garden into different beds and give the beds diverse looks as described above. However, the center of all these beds should be the focal point for the entire garden. The center should shout the most and give the garden its personality. You could use a simple birdbath design that works well for bird and bee plants in a flower garden. To make sure that the garden remains alive throughout the year, use annual plants at the center of your garden. The annual herbs will ensure that even if the rest of the garden sheds, there is still some beauty to be seen.

## DECIDING WHAT TO PLANT WHERE

Planning a garden is all about deciding what to plant and where to plant it. As you can see from the plan guide above, some factors guide us into deciding what to plant and where to plant. Although you may want to plant some herbs that I have not recommended, you should make your choices well. When deciding what to plant and where to plant, there are some key factors to consider.

## THE CLIMATE ZONE

The first thing you should consider before choosing to plant an herb is its climate zone. Some plants will not do well in certain zones. Even if you provide the best care, you may still not be able to grow in your zone. First, check the climate zone of the herb you are about to plant. Some herbs are generally tolerant of most climates. For example, chives do well in most climate zones, starting from 3 - 9. On the contrary, nasturtium only thrives in climate zones 6-9). If you are going to choose between these two herbs, you should consider the climate zone where you live and the possibility of nurturing the herb to maturity.

The other option you have is to provide an ideal environment for your herb outside its growing zone. Some grow the herbs in-house or in greenhouse gardens with custom climates. If you can create the ideal temperature and environment for the herb, you may go ahead and plant it in your garden.

## THE AVERAGE HEIGHT OF THE HERB

The other factor to look at is the height of the herb. There those who only want to plant short herbs that will stay at ground level. If you are looking to create a garden at the grass level, avoid herbs that mature into trees with long stems and branches. When considering such factors, you should factor in the size of your garden. Those who have large gardens can comfortably plant herbs that mature to more than 3 feet high. However, if you have limited space but you wish to grow some herbs, settle for those that don't grow past 3 feet.

## THE MATURITY PERIOD

The other factor to look at is the maturity period of the herbs. There are some herbs that will mature in just a few months, while others will take several years. If you are looking for herbs you can harvest often and use, you should go for ones that mature fast. If you are looking for herbs that will stay around for the longest time possible, you could settle for ones that take time to mature. With that said, herbal gardening should be a continuous venture. Once you get started, you should continue growing and propagating your herbs. Even if one herb matures in just 3 months, you should find a way of replanting so that you always have a constant supply of the herb.

## HARVESTING PERIOD

Besides maturity, you need to look at the bloom and harvesting period. The flowering period helps you determine the look of your garden. Most gardeners use the bloom period of flowers to decide the pattern of the garden. For instance, instead of planting flowers that bloom at the same time in one garden, you could combine flowers with different bloom periods. This way, the garden is always alive, even at the time when the flowers are not blooming. For instance, Italian Parsley blooms in spring while calendula blooms in mid-summer. Having these flowers in one garden will mean that your garden will remain lively right from summer to the end of spring.

Most importantly, you should consider the tolerance of the herbs you are planting. Some herbs can tolerate harsh climates, pests, and poor soils, while others require critical care. If you do not have plenty of time on your hands, it is advisable to stick to tolerant herbs. Most of the tolerant herbs may survive out of the prescribed climate zone. For instance, parsley is prescribed for climate zones 12-15, but we grow it in climate zone 6. This shows how well tolerant herbs work. Some of the most tolerant herbs you should consider include mint, dill, parsley, sorrel, chives, coriander, sorrel, and lovage. There are many tolerant herbs that you should consider, especially if you live far north.

## ACCESSIBILITY

Lastly, when choosing the herbs to plant in your herb garden, consider their accessibility. In other words, do not fill your garden with herbs that are easily accessible locally. When I started herbal gardening, I would plant all types of herbs I came across. After some time, I started getting rid of commercially accessible herbs. If you can easily buy some herbs from the market, there is no need to fill your garden. Try planting herbs that are not readily available. However, you are also allowed to plant herbs that are accessible elsewhere as long as you have a large backyard. If you have sufficient space to plant all types of herbs, go ahead and factor in as many herbs as possible. However, if you have limited garden space, try sticking to the herbs that are important and inaccessible.

## THE TOP 25 HERBAL PLANTS FOR YOUR GARDEN

Although there are plenty of plants you can grow in your garden, we will not review all the plants you can grow. I have selected 25 of the most potent herbs that can be grown in your backyard. These herbs are tolerant and do not require much attention. Most importantly, they are potent with healing compounds and can treat almost all diseases that affect humanity. For the rest of the book, we will focus on growing, maturing, and preparing these herbs for their medicinal value. Here are the top 25 plants to consider for your backyard herbal garden.

**Rosemary**: Rosemary is one of the most potent herbal plants to grow in your garden. Officially known as Salvia Rosmarinus, the plant is a woody perennial with fragrant evergreen leaves. It blooms with white, pink, blue, and purple flowers. The flower is native to Mediterranean regions and is used to treat various diseases, including indigestion, vomiting, and nausea, among others. The herb thrives in climate zones 5 to 8, but it is only perennial in climate zones 6 and 7.

**Basil**: Basil is another of the most common herbs that are grown in backyard gardens. Basil thrives in pots and containers as opposed to planting directly in the soil. This herb is known for its culinary and medicinal benefits. It is native to Asia and central Africa. Still, it can also be grown in the US and other parts of North America. The herb thrives in soil with a pH of 5.1 to 5.8 and can do well in climate zones 2 - 11. However, it is only perennial in climate zones 10 and 11.

Basil is used for treating many conditions, including stomach spasms, loss of appetite, intestinal gas, kidney conditions, fluid retention, head colds, and mild infections, among others.

**Cayenne**: Cayenne is one of the most commonly used herbs due to its culinary benefits. This herb is tolerant to most climates and should be present in every herbal garden. The hot and beautiful red pepper makes the right decoration for your garden and food as well. Although the pepper can grow in climate zones 6 to 11, it is perennial in zones 9 to 11. This herb is used to treat blood circulatory problems, stop bleeding, and stop or slow heart attacks.

**Aloe Vera**: Aloe vera is one of the most common and popular herbal medicines in the world. Some herbalists refer to aloe vera as a cure-all herb, although such remarks do not have scientific backing. This succulent is evergreen and originates from the Arabian Peninsula. However, it grows well in tropical, semitropical, and arid climates. Aloe vera does not thrive in cold climates, but you can cultivate the herb if you reside in climate zones 10 to 11. It should be grown in regions where temperatures stay above 30 F. Aloe vera can treat a lot of conditions, including burns, digestive problems, and acne, among others.

**Burdock**: Burdock is a perennial plant that acts as one of the most beneficial herbs. This herb belongs to the family Asteraceae and is native to Europe and Asia. However, the herb can grow in some parts of North America. Although the herb may not thrive in all parts of America, it grows in climate zones 6 - 8. However, it thrives best in climate zone 8.

Burdock is taken to increase urine flow, reduce bacteria in the body, and reduce fevers. The herb is also claimed to treat colds and even reduce the risk of cancer. Although certain claims do not have scientific backing, there is no harm in trying out this natural herb.

**Goldenseal**: Goldenseal is also one of the commonly cultivated herbs at home. Also known as orange root or yellow puccoon, this herb is ideal for backyard farming due to its tolerance to harsh climates. It belongs to the family *Ranunculaceae* and is native to Southern Canada. It is easily recognized by its thick, yellow, knotted roots.

According to the US department of agriculture, this herb can be grown in climate zones 2 to 11, but it is only perennial in zones 3 to 8.

Goldenseal is used to treat common colds and other upper respiratory conditions. It is also used to treat digestive disorders, including stomach pain and swellings, peptic ulcers, diarrhea, and colitis, among other conditions.

**Calendula**: Calendula is one of my favorite herbs due to the diversity of its uses. Furthermore, it blooms with sunny yellow or orange flowers that light up the garden. If you are in a dilemma about the herb to place at the center of your garden, try working with calendula. This herb is tolerant to most climates and thrives in the summer just about anywhere. This flower is a product of garden breeding but is often referred to as being native to the eastern United States. The herb can be grown in climate zones 2 to 11, but it is only perennial in zones 9 to 11. It thrives during summers in zones 7 to 11.

Calendula is used to treat a variety of diseases, including sore throats, menstrual cramps, duodenal, and to prevent cancer. The herb is also used to prevent muscle spasms, reduce fever, and start menstrual periods.

**Chickweed**: Chickweed is one of the few herbs that are entirely misunderstood. Although most people bypass chickweed every day, it offers plenty of medicinal benefits. Chickweed is not necessarily cultivated but can be allowed to grow. The herb usually appears during the cooler temperatures and dies in the late spring. It thrives at temperatures between 53 and 63 degrees F. Although it grows naturally, it can help beautify your garden during early spring. With its beautiful multicolored flowers, it should be more readily grown.

Chickweed is used in reducing inflammation and treating most inflammatory conditions. It is also used to fight germs and promote weight loss.

**Chamomile:** The other herb that is commonly grown in backyard gardens is chamomile. The health benefits of chamomile cannot be overemphasized. This herb has diverse uses right from the kitchen to your medicinal needs. It is recognized by its honey scent and sweet taste.

Chamomile can be grown in all climate zones in the US through division or by direct seeds. However, the herb thrives in climate zones 3 to 9. Such a vast growing zone just indicates the tolerance of the herb. It is one of the herbs that need little maintenance.

Chamomile is used to treat many diseases, including hay fever, muscle spasms, menstrual disorders, gastrointestinal disorders, rheumatic pain, hemorrhoids, ulcers, and insomnia, among others. The essential oil made from this herb is used in cosmetics for skincare.

**Feverfew**: Feverfew is another beautiful garden herb thanks to its all-white flowers. The herb has more to offer than just beauty. It treats many conditions and is also tolerant to most climates and soil types. Although this herb is native to South-Eastern Europe, it grows in most regions in North America. It does well in climate zones 3 to 10, but it thrives in zones 5 to 10.

Feverfew gets its name from its medicinal benefits of reducing fevers. Besides the treatment of fevers, the herb is also used to reduce or stop migraines, toothaches, stomach aches, rheumatoid arthritis, reduce labor during childbirth, treat infertility, and insect bites, among others. This beautiful flower is one of the most diverse herbs and can be grown in most regions in America.

**Dandelion**: Dandelions are only known for their decorative purposes in gardens. However, besides their bright yellow flowers, dandelions also have many health benefits to offer. Due to its brightness, dandelions should always be planted in a multi-colored bed. Although dandelions quickly crop up like weeds in your gardens, you may also wish to cultivate them. They are non-native invasive weeds that quickly spread during spring. However, you can preserve their seeds to keep them from going away. Dandelions thrive in moist climate zones in the US and Canada. You can grow them in zones 3 to 10 for the best outcome. Dandelions are potent anti-inflammatories and antioxidants. They can also help reduce blood pressure, blood sugar, and regulate cholesterol levels in the body.

**Lavender**: This is one of the most common flowers in most gardens. Lavender is a beautiful flower with a wonderful smell. It attracts bees and butterflies due to its remarkable scent and appearance. However, it also has so many health benefits. The beautiful purple flower can grow in most conditions but thrives in well-draining soil under warm conditions. In the US, the flower can be grown in most climates but thrives in hardiness zone 5. Lavender treats many conditions, and its essential oil is used as an antiseptic and anti-inflammatory. Due to these properties, lavender oil is often used to treat inflammatory skin conditions and reduce bacterial infections. Lavender teas and concoctions can also be used to treat anxiety, insomnia, depression, and restlessness, among other conditions.

**Ginger:** Ginger is one of the most beneficial herbs you can plant in your garden. This sweet and spicy herb is a rhizome and not a root, as many people believe. The herb is an excellent additive to tea and fermented foods and also acts as a spice in recipes.

Ginger can be grown in some parts of the US and takes about 10 months to mature. The stem and leaves are dark green and will remain green throughout until it's time to harvest. Ginger does not thrive in every zone but does well in zone 7.

Ginger is used in treating various conditions, including colds, nausea, arthritis, migraines, and hypertension. The herb is also anti-inflammatory and increases the flow of blood in the body. The herb also helps in reducing flatulence and stomach issues such as diarrhea and nausea.

**Garlic**: Garlic is another of the best all-round medicinal herbs with plenty of uses. Garlic can be grown in most zones and soil types and is tolerant to pests. With that said, if you wish to grow garlic in your garden, you have to get the timing right. In hardiness zones, 3-5, garlic should be planted during the months of September and October. Plant your garlic between early September and October so that they are out of the ground by December. In climate zones 5 - 7, you should plant the garlic in late October. In climate zones 7-9, you can plant in October to November. In zones 9 to 10, you should plant in late October to November. If you do not get the timing right, you may end up messing with the growth of the plant.

Garlic is used to treat colds and coughs. It is also used to boost the immune system, treat asthma, and manage heart disease. Some people also use garlic to manage pain caused by arthritis or toothaches.

**Yarrow**: Yarrow is one of the most beautiful backyard garden herbs. This herb grows in bunches of feathery grayish leaves that can easily be recognized. Besides the beautiful leaves, yarrow also has plenty of health benefits. This herb is native to the disturbed soils of prairies and meadows. In the Northern Hemisphere, the herb thrives on the edges of forests. The herb -which produces white flowers-, can grow up to 36 inches in the ideal environment. In the US, it can be grown in climate zones 3 to 9; however, it does well in zones 8 and 9.

The herb has been traditionally used to induce sweating, stop bleeding, reduce heavy menstrual flow, reduce menstrual pain, relieve GI ailments, lower high blood pressure, improve circulation, and tone varicose veins.

**Valerian**: This is another beautiful flowering plant that can be cultivated in backyard gardens. It grows to about 4 feet tall and produces clusters of lacy white flowers. Besides the beauty it adds to your garden, it will benefit your family with its medicinal components. There are more than 2000 varieties of valerian, which means that some strains may not be favorable in all climates. The plant is perennial in zone 4, although it can grow well in zones 2 to 9. It prefers a balance of warm climates and cool shades. The herb is native to Europe and China but can be cultivated in the US.

Valerian is a strong sedative that is used to induce sleep, reduce anxiety and stress. There are more studies underway to discover other uses of the herb.

**Thyme**: Thyme is one of the herbs that every gardener must grow. Thyme is beautiful and has a sweet scent that attracts bees and butterflies. It is also tolerant of most soil types hence easy to cultivate even for beginners. Although it can grow in the US and other parts of North America, it does not fare well in cold winters. The herb will thrive in hardiness zone 5 but can be grown through to zone 10. However, in higher zones such as 10 and 9, more care should be taken. Due to its sweet scent, thyme is used as a relaxant. It is also used to treat coughs and other upper respiratory conditions. Some studies have suggested that it can be used to treat bronchitis.

**St. John's Wort**: St. John's Wort is one of the most popular herbs due to its medicinal value. This herb can grow in all soil types and can be grown in some parts of the US. It does well in hardiness zones 5 to 6, although some people grow it in zones 7 to 10. This herb acts as a potent antidepressant and can treat symptoms associated with depression such as nervousness, tiredness, poor appetite, and trouble sleeping. It can also help manage some symptoms of mental and personality disorders.

**Plantain**: Plantain is one of the easiest herbs to grow. In most parts of the US, it can thrive with minimal care. Plantain belongs to the family of bananas and is believed to have originated from Southeast Asia. With that being said, the herb cannot survive in regions with extremely cold temperatures. It needs about 10 to 15 months without freezing temperatures to start flowering. If you reside in hardiness zones 8 to 11, you can comfortably mature some plantain in your backyard.

When it comes to medicinal value, plantain is one of the most potent herbs. It is used to treat various conditions, including cough, wounds, inflamed skin, and insect bites. Its leaves are also crushed and used to treat insect bites and skin infections, among other uses.

**Peppermint**: Peppermint is one of the fast-spreading perennial herbs. It usually takes over the garden and may end up overpowering other crops in your garden. However, it can be contained with proper management. This herb is known for its spicy, pungent scent and can be recognized from a distance. Peppermint is grown within climate zones 3 to 8 and is perennial in most regions. This herb is used to treat flatulence, menstrual pains, diarrhea, nausea, and anxiety.

**Oregano**: Oregano is another herb that can be planted within your garden. The beauty of this herb is that it grows well once you have it in the soil. The plant originates from Southern and Easter Eurasia and belongs to the mint family. Oregano is used as a spice in most Mexican, Spanish and Italian dishes. It is a hardy perennial plant that can grow in most backyard gardens.

Although it can grow in most climate zones in the US and Canada, it mainly thrives in hardiness zones 5 to 10.

Oregano herbs have plenty of health and dietary benefits, including fighting bacterial infections, reducing viral infections, and decreasing inflammation, among other uses.

**Mullein:** Mullein is a powerful home garden herb that most people just assume to be a regular weed. This weed sometimes grows into a tall stalk as high as 7 feet. It is usually covered with yellow flowers in the summer. Due to its climatic requirements, it does not thrive in most parts of North America. It requires full sun and lots of water. If you live in mountainous areas, you may grow mullein in creek beds. Although it's not commonly cultivated due to its water needs, it is worth trying due to its various health benefits. Mullein is believed to have originated from the Eurasia regions only brought to the US by early settlers. The plant is perennial and grows in USDA hardiness zones 3 to 9; however, it thrives in zones 8 to 9.

The main reason for including this herb on this list is the diversity of its health benefits. Mullein can be used to treat cough, tuberculosis, bronchitis, pneumonia, earaches, colds, hoarseness, chills, flu, fever, allergies, swine flu, tonsillitis, and sore throat. Other uses include asthma, diarrhea, colic, gastrointestinal bleeding, migraines, joint pain, and gout.

**Marshmallow Root**: Marshmallow root is another herb that you could cultivate in your backyard. Although this herb is not commonly cultivated by most gardeners, I love it due to the health benefits it has to offer. The herb is tolerant to most soils and climates and can be grown within most areas in the US. According to the US Agricultural Department, the tree can be grown in climate zones 3 to 9, where it thrives in sunny but cold climates. It can also be grown on the edges of mash land and grassy banks of lakes. If you live in a region with abundant water sources, you can cultivate marshmallow root without a problem. Marshmallow roots are the potent medicinal part of the tree. The roots are used to treat various conditions, including inflammation of the digestive tract. Several studies have also suggested that extracts from the roots can be used to treat irritated mucous membranes.

**Lemon Balm:** The last herb you should consider planting in your garden is lemon balm. This is one of my favorite herbs due to the ease of maintenance. The herb grows almost everywhere and does not have strict maintenance routines. Lemon balm belongs to the mint family and has a pleasant scent. Although the plant can be cultivated in semi-outdoor environments, it thrives outdoors. It can be cultivated in the United States in hardiness zones 4 to 9. According to the US Department of Agriculture, this herb needs winter mulch and well-drained sandy soil to survive.

This herb offers various health benefits, including management of stress and anxiety, promotes sleep, improves appetite, and treats discomfort and indigestion, just to mention a few. It is commonly used in teas and other beverages due to the ease of preparation.

There are many types of planters you may use in your gardening. The planter you chose depends on the type of plants you are growing. Some plants have long roots that need to take depth. When planting such herbs in your garden, try to use vertical planters or plant in garden beds. If you are planting crops with shallow roots, you may utilize planters that do not allow penetration of roots. Planters are categorized based on their form, size, and material of manufacture. In this section, we are going to look at three main types of planters and the herbs they are suited for. We will categorize our planters based on their form/shape. The main aim is to determine the crops that do well in planters versus those that require to be planted in garden beds directly. From the list of herbs above, we have those that grow tall to over 7 feet. Such herbs cannot be planted in planters since the roots will overgrow the depth of most planters. For such, we have the option of using the natural bed or customized planters. For the sake of this book, we will look at three types of planters: Box, vertical, and bed planters.

Box planters are usually made with a square or rectangular base. Such boxes are ideal for herbs that do not have long roots. They are also ideal for plants that are non-spreading. In the list of our herbs above, we can grow the shallow-rooted herbs in box planters. Some of the herbs that do well in box planters include basil, aloe vera, goldenseal, burdock, among others. Most of the shorter herbs that do not mature past 3 feet tall can comfortably be grown in box planters. With that said, you should consider several factors when growing your herbs in box planters. If you are growing an herb that has relatively long roots such as aloe vera, you should use a box planter of significant height. Most box planters are usually limited in height and width. Depending on whether the herb has spreading roots or vertical roots, choose a planter that works.

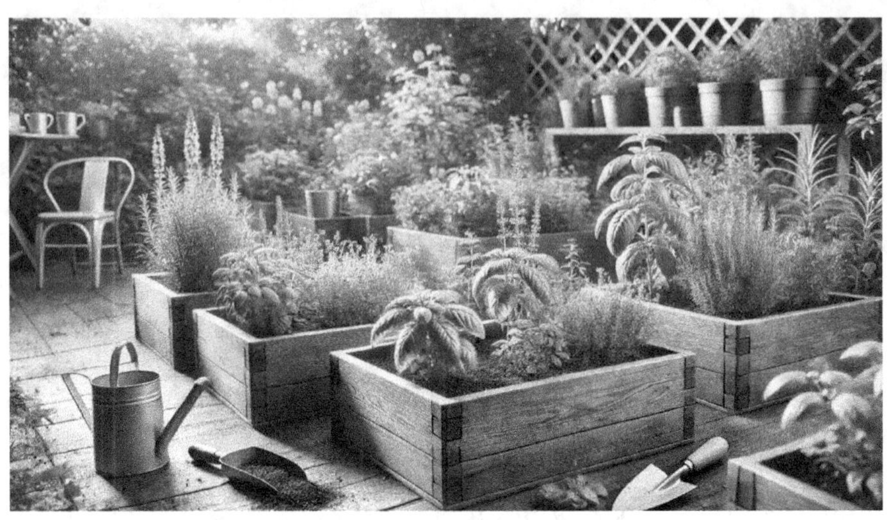

In some situations, you may love the idea of planting your herbs in box planters even though they may not be ideal for box planters. In such cases, you can customize your boxes to allow you to plant your herbs comfortably. For instance, if you are growing herbs with deep-reaching roots, such as mullein, you have to modify the base of the box so that the roots can easily penetrate into the garden bed. If you are planting herbs with spreading roots, you could make the planter much wider than an average box to accommodate the spreading roots.

The other type of planters used in farming herbs is the vertical garden planters. Most vertical planters are designed to have sufficient vertical highlights. Such planters are usually not ideal for plants that have long roots. They are used by individuals who have carpeted backyards but desire to grow some root spreading herbs.

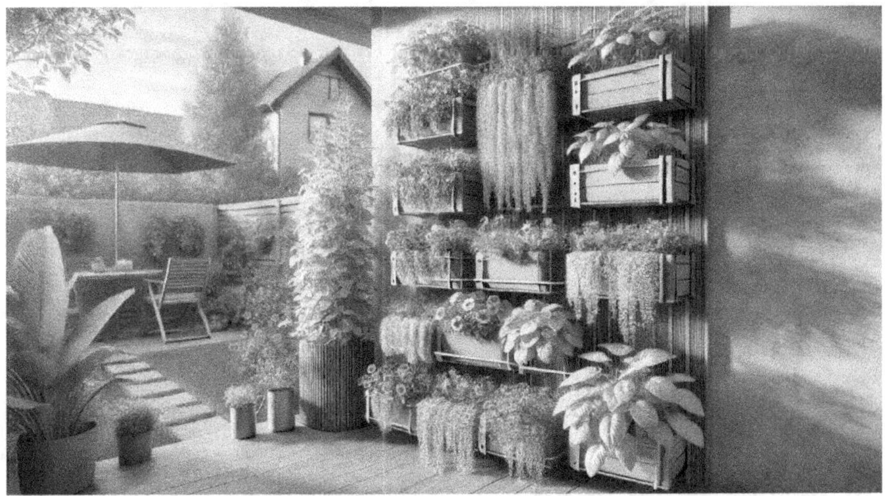

While vertical planters are ideal for crops with spreading roots, they are not stable enough to hold very tall plants. You should keep in mind that a vertical planter is already elevated. If you were to plant an herb that grows to 7 feet, the planters would easily get unstable and topple. Therefore, such vertical planters are ideal for plants with long roots but shorter stems. Some herbs you may grow in the vertical planters include yarrow, roses, feverfew, and dandelion, among others. Although some of these plants don't necessarily have long roots, they have a beautiful look on vertical planters. With that in mind, make sure your vertical planter has the ideal surface for holding herbs that have spreading roots.

## GARDEN BEDS

Lastly, we can plant our herbs in garden beds. Garden beds present the ideal growing situation for most herbs. This is because garden beds allow the herbs to grow their roots to the maximum. However, garden beds present various challenges. Most garden beds may not have the ideal soil for your desired herb. If the soil is acid, yet your plant requires alkaline soil, you will have to invest a lot of money on treating the soil to attain the required conditions. Besides the condition of the soil, garden beds also present the challenge of pests, weeds, and season changes. During the freezing winters, you cannot uproot an herb planted in the garden and keep it indoors. With planter herbs, you can easily transfer the vessel inside to protect your herbs from cold weather.

Garden beds are ideal for herbs that have long roots or tall stems. For instance, plantains can grow to between 7 and 30 feet tall. For such a huge tree, you cannot plant within any type of planter. Such trees take longer to mature and have their roots penetrate deep. You can only plant them directly into the soil. Even if you wish to start it in planters, the planter should have an open base to allow the roots to penetrate to the ground.

## UNDERSTANDING CLIMATE ZONES

When planting medicinal herbs, you should consider your climate zone. Climate zones help determine the possibility of a particular crop doing well in a given region. The United States Department of Agriculture USDA categorizes the entire country into different climatic zones. Hardiness zones help determine the suitability of a specified location when growing individual plants. The

USDA provides a hardiness zone map that can be used to determine which crops to plant in your garden.

The USDA plant hardiness map shown below can help you determine the zone where to plant your crops and the ideal temperature for the crops. As we have seen in the sections above, each herb has a specific zone in which it thrives. For instance, we have established that chives can do well in most zones, starting from zone 2 to 12. However, the herb is only perennial in zones 9 to 11. Hardiness zones represent a region on the map where certain crops do well. The map of hardiness is categorized in numbers, starting with 1 to 15. The lower the hardiness numbers, the colder the region. Zones 1 and 2 are too cold to support the growth of most herbs. As a result, such regions experience little to no agricultural activities. The higher you go in terms of hardiness figures, the hotter it gets. Very hot areas in the hardiness zones 13 to14 are also very hostile to most plants. In general, herbs and their crops thrive in hardiness zone 3 to 12. In these sections, most of the herbs can be grown comfortably.

To determine your hardiness zone, you have to look at the map provided by the USDA. Have a look at the map below, find your location, and determine the hardiness zone. After determining your zone, compare with the hardiness zone of the herb you wish to plant. In the section above, we have indicated the hardiness zones for each of the 25 herbs listed. Do not plant herbs that fall outside your zone by a large margin.

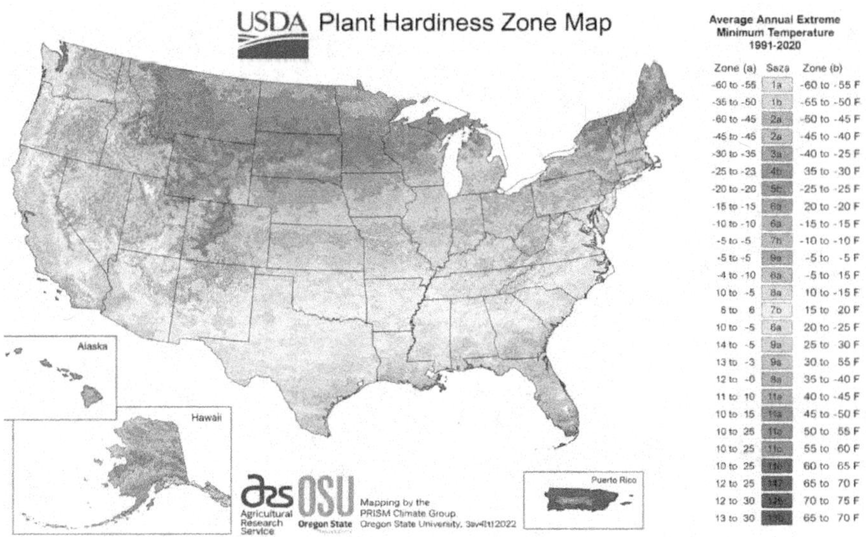


As you can see from the map, the zones are primarily divided based on the temperature. The minimum annual temperature is divided into 10 degrees F zones. If you cannot find your location accurately, check out the USDA

website
(https://planthardiness.ars.usda.gov/PHZMWeb/) to
determine your exact climate zone providing your zip
code. The system provides highly accurate figures that
will help you determine your exact hardiness zone.

# Chapter 3: How to Grow Medicinal Herbs

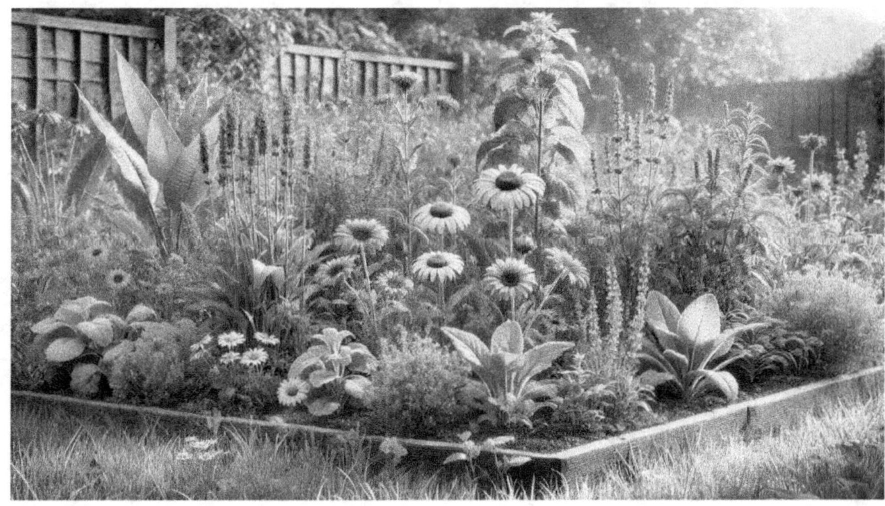

When it comes to growing herbs, each plant has specific growing requirements. You should consider the requirements of each herb in terms of sunlight, soil, water, and fertilizer. Some herbs will require well-aerated soil, while others will need soil that can retain water. In either case, you should find a way of providing the best conditions for your herbs. If you are planting an herb that requires plenty of water, make sure you provide the water sufficiently. We are going to look at the water, soil, sunlight, and fertilizer needs of our herbs and try categorizing the herbs that can be planted together based on such needs.

## WATER REQUIREMENTS FOR HERBS

First, you need to determine the herbs that require plenty of water from your list of chosen herbs. In general, we categorize our herbs' water needs per week. If you plant your herbs in planters, you can gauge how much water the plant takes every week. By using a medium-sized box planter, we categorize plants that require less than 1 inch of water per week are being drought resistant. From our list of 25 herbs above, some herbs can thrive on less than 1 inch of water per week. These include aloe vera, dandelions, yarrows, thyme, and St. John's Wort. These plants require watering just once per week but will not die if you miss the schedule.

The second category contains the plants that require about 1 inch to 1.5 inches of water per week. These are categorized as average water users and must be watered once every week. From our list of 25 herbs to plant, the plants that require daily watering include basil, rosemary, goldenseal, calendula, feverfew, mullein, and marshmallow. These plants do not require too much water but should be kept moist throughout.

The third category includes those that require more than 2 inches of water weekly. These are high demand herbs that should only be planted by those who have time to water throughout. Among the high water demand herbs on this list are valerian, plantain, and cayenne. However, some of these herbs can only be watered once per week and will thrive.

## SOIL REQUIREMENTS

The other factor to consider when growing your plants is their soil demands. There are those that require acidic soil- where the pH is less than 7, while others require alkaline soil, where the pH is greater than 7. Although some herbs require acidic conditions, they are just a few. Most of the herbs on this list will do well in alkaline soil except for Oregano, peppermint, chives, basil, and thyme.

These herbs should be grown in soils with a pH between 5.5 and 7.0. However, you can still mature all of these herbs in soils with a pH between 7 and 7.5. The rest of the herbs on this list do well in alkaline soils.

Besides the pH of the soil, the other factor you should consider is the ability of the soil to drain/retain water. Some herbs generally do well in soils that are well aerated while others work well for soils that are water retaining. In our garden, we generally grow our herbs in loam soil. Such soil has an average water retaining rate and can work well for most herbs. However, for herbs that need less than 1 inch of water, you may choose to plant them in well-draining sandy soil. Whether you grow your crop in sandy or loamy soil depends on its water retention.

## SUNLIGHT EXPOSURE

The other important factor you have to consider when planting your herbs is their sun exposure requirements. Some herbs will only grow under full sunlight exposure, while others can even grow in a dark room. The sunlight exposure demands of a crop determine the possibility of planting it indoors.

All the herbs on this list thrive in full sunlight; however, some of the herbs are delicate and require some shade during their early days. If you choose to plant direct seeds into the garden, ensure that they are under the shade. When most crops are young, they should be grown under partial sunlight. This way, you reduce the chances of crop weathering in the sun.

With that said, the sun exposure demands of most herbs are almost the same. Most herbs need to be exposed to direct light for at least 4 hours per day. However, if you live in a place that is too hot, you should avoid delicate herbs such as garlic and calendula. You should go for herbs that are more tolerant to hot temperatures and less water.

Among the herbs on this list, you can plant basil, chives, rosemary, oregano, aloe vera, and peppermint indoors with partial exposure to light. However, some flowers such as basil can be grown completely indoors as long as you provide artificial lighting.



# FERTILIZER NEEDS

The fertilizer needs of these herbs differ depending on the soil in which you plant the herbs. For instance, if you plant herbs that require alkaline soil in acid soil, you have to use a more alkaline fertilizer such as ammonium sulfate to balance the quality of the soil. With that said, it is not absolutely necessary to use fertilizer when planting most of these herbs. Some of the herbs can simply be planted in the ideal soil without adding extra fertilizer. The best option for gardeners is to use homemade manure, such as compost of chicken poop. Such waste usually balances the soil pretty well to avoid the complications associated with fertilization. We have categorized the plants on our list, depending on their fertilizer needs.

The first group includes those that require less or no fertilizer at all. Most of the herbs that are categorized as having less or none for fertilizer need are tolerant of most soil types. Among those that can survive with little or no fertilizer include yarrows, St. John's Wort, Dandelions, aloe vera, and burdocks. Such herbs can easily grow without the need to fertilize.

The second category of plants includes those that require medium fertilization. These are herbs that can survive with manure or basic calcium or phosphorus fertilizer. However, the main idea for the medium fertilization crops is to ensure that the soil requirements are met. If the crop does well in acidic aerated soil, just ensure that you plant in soil that meets the definition, and you will have little problems in regard to its fertilizer needs. Some of the crops with medium fertilization needs include basil, rosemary, thyme, and mullein.

The third category of crops to consider includes those that have high fertilization needs. There are some crops that demand nutrients and must be fertilized to thrive. These are crops that will have to be supplied with some fertilizer at least once or twice within the season. Some of the plants that have high nutritional needs on this list include garlic, cayenne pepper, dandelions, marshmallow, and plantain. The fertilization needs of plantain are too high, and those who choose to farm must be careful. The crop requires a regular supply of nitrous fertilizer to thrive.

## PLANTS THAT GROW WELL TOGETHER

When categorizing herbs that grow well together, there are many factors to consider. In our categorization in the first chapter, we were looking at the desired appearance of the garden. If your aim is to grow a beautiful garden, you may arrange your herbs according to their looks, the blooming seasons, and the food/water needs. It is usually not easy to choose the herbs to grow together for those who are just starting. You should not only look at the beauty of the herbs or the height. You must consider the fertilizer, water, and sun exposure needs of all the herbs.

I have categorized some of the plants that you can grow together as follows.

Rosemary is one of the herbs that have fewer demands. As we have seen, the herb can be planted with minimum fertilizer and water. The herb grows in zones 5 to 12 and thrives in zone 7. The other herbs that can be grown under similar conditions include Oregano, thyme, lavender, and sage. Since all these herbs do not grow too tall and do not have a woody stem, they can be grown together without any trouble.

## PLANTS TO GROW WITH BASIL

Basil requires relatively medium levels of fertilizer, about 1 inch of water per week, and full sun exposure or limited shade. In other words, the herb can be grown outdoors and indoors as long as you provide the right amount of moisture. It thrives in loamy soil and does well in zones 2 to 11. In other words, it can thrive in most regions throughout the US. This herb can be grown together with parsley, cilantro, Aragon, and thyme.

This herb does not have strict requirements since it thrives in most soil types. It can grow within zone 2- 11 and requires sufficient sun exposure. This herb can grow well with herbs such as lemon thyme, aloe vera, burdock, peppermint, and cayenne pepper, among others.

## PLANTS TO GROW WITH CALENDULA

Since calendula blooms well in cooler weather with low humidity, it should be combined with similar herbs. It can be grown with feverfew, chickweed, and other herbs that flourish in spring. With that said, you should consider the water and fertilizer needs of these herbs.

The other way of combining herbs when growing is to look at the height of the mature tree. For instance, plantain may grow all the way to 30 feet high. This means that it can be grown with other herbs that do not need full sun exposure. If you are planting delicate herbs that must be protected from direct sunshine, plant them directly below your plantain tree to reduce their exposure to sunshine.

Lastly, consider the soil drainage and the planters you are using. If you are planting herbs that use the same type of soil, for instance, marshmallow and aloe vera require almost similar soil types. They thrive in well-drained soil. Such plants can be planted together as long as one does not overpower the other in terms of water and nutrient consumption.

## DEALING WITH WEEDS AND PESTS

Herbs are supposed to be harvested and used at any time. For this reason, you should avoid using pesticides on your herbs as much as possible. Some pesticides may contain harmful components that are not ideal for human consumption. It is advisable to use alternative methods of dealing with weeds and pests. Some of the ways to deal with weeds and pests include:

### REMOVE WEEDS BY HAND

The best way of dealing with weeds is to remove them by hand. This way, you reduce the chances of poisoning your herbs with harmful pesticides. However, pulling weeds with your hands does require effort. You have to work hard to ensure that the weeds do not grow beyond manageable levels. With this approach, you will have to keep a close eye on the herbs and pull out the weeds as soon as they start growing.

## Use Companion Herbs

Some crops naturally repel pests. If you do not want to use chemical pesticides, you could plant such crops alongside your herbs to repel the harmful pests. For instance, you may grow your thyme with marigolds or roses with garlic. Garlic is a natural repellent to most insects and will reduce the chances of your garden getting infected.

## Pick Insects by Hand

The other option is to drive out insects by picking them. Although this approach might be tiresome, it can work if you have plenty of time on your hands. You will have to be watchful such that the insects are picked before they start spreading. The best way is to pluck out leaves and branches that are infected before the insects start spreading to other leaves and crops in your garden.

## USE BEER TRAPS

Slugs and snails are attracted to the smell of beer. If you have plenty of snails in your garden, you can create a beer trap to capture them all. Just put some beer in an open dish and allow it to stay within your garden overnight. You will find some slugs and snails trapped within.

## COVER YOUNG PLANTS AT NIGHT

The other option when dealing with pests is to cover your plants at night. Although this approach is usually discouraged because plants need oxygen, you can cover them using a porous material. Use a material that resembles a porous mosquito net to cover the young plants to reduce the chances of being attacked by insects. Most insects crawl at night and disappear into hiding during the day. By covering your young plants at night, you reduce the chances of the crops being attacked by insects. However, this approach cannot protect your crops from all insects. It will be effective against larger insects, but the smaller ones may find a way through.

## ATTRACT LADYBUGS AND BIRDS

The other option is to use predators to control pests. This is the best approach for those who are engaged in multipurpose backyard farming. For instance, if you grow herbs in the garden and also keep birds such as chickens, you could use your birds to deal with the pests. With that said, chickens usually feed on large pests such as snails and grasshoppers. You should encourage insect predators such as ladybugs to thrive in your garden too. This way, the ladybugs control the microorganisms while the birds at home control the population of larger insects.

## KEEP YOUR GARDEN CLEAN

The best way to deal with pests and weeds without necessarily using pesticides is by keeping your garden clean. Ensure that the area around your crops is clean and without weeds. The garden will not have pests as long as there are no weeds. However, if you allow weeds to grow around the herbs, they will start attracting pests. Furthermore, weeds compete for food with your herbs, making it difficult for your herbs to thrive. With that said, the work of maintaining a clean garden isn't easy. You have to keep your eyes open and ensure that you carry out weekly maintenance routines.

## USE NATURAL REMEDIES

The other option is to use natural remedies to drive away pests. For instance, you could spray some ash within the farm to drive away pests. Many natural remedies could be used to drive away pests, without necessarily using pesticides. Other remedies that can be used include table salt, vinegar, insect repellent plants such as garlic, among others. Such natural remedies are less costly and will keep your garden clean without the risk of causing chemical poisoning.

## HARVESTING

Each of the plants listed in this book has a specific method of harvesting. For plants that we use leaves, the harvesting process is as simple as plucking the leaves. For plants that include harvesting the stem or roots, you have to get rid of the entire plant during harvesting. For plants where we harvest the fruits, it's much easier since you only pluck the fruits. With that said, you should be very careful when dealing with each plant since some are very delicate. The harvesting process should not mean that the entire farm has to be cleaned away. Let us look at the approaches applied to harvest each of the listed plants.

**Basil**: To harvest basil, you have to pluck a few leaves from each section of the plant. Make sure you do not cut off the stems. Harvesting the leaves encourages the basil to grow more.

**Rosemary**: For rosemary, we harvest sprigs instead of leaves. To harvest, cut off about 2 to 3 inches of each spring, leaving green leaves behind. Do not cut the sprig too close to the roots. This will allow the flower to continue growing.

**Cayenne**: For cayenne, you have to wait until the peppers are mature before you harvest. Although you may harvest them green, wait until they are turning red. Pluck the fruit from its branches and use it accordingly.

**Aloe Vera**: For aloe vera, we harvest the thick succulent leaves. To harvest the herb, use a sharp knife to cut one leaf close to the stem. Do not cut too many leaves from the same plant since you need it to recover. Just cut 1 to 3 leaves from every plant while harvesting.

**Burdock**: For burdock, harvesting entails uprooting the entire plant to collect the roots. Since the roots are not easy to uproot, you will need special tools to uproot your plant. You will also need to be careful not to cut through the roots when uprooting. Dig around the main stalk with a shovel until you see the roots. Cut them with a sharp knife and wash.

**Goldenseal**: Harvesting goldenseal is a pretty simple process. Since the roots are very shallow, the harvesting process involves plucking the crop from the ground. To ensure that all the roots come out, hold the crop close to the ground, and gently lift it up. Wash off the mud and use the roots accordingly.

**Calendula**: For the case of calendula, we harvest the petals of the flower. Once the flowers start to bloom, you should be ready to harvest your herbs. To harvest, pluck the flower head gently using your hand or a pair of scissors. You should only harvest the ones you wish to use at the time.

**Chickweed**: For chickweed, you may either harvest the flowers or the stem and some leaves. The ideal harvesting option is to cut the top part of freshly growing weeds. Cut about 2 to 23 inches of the fresh herb using a pair of scissors.

**Chamomile**: Chamomile is harvested in the morning just before the dew dries. To harvest, pick the flower that has just opened up just below the stalk. Once you have the flower, pop off the stalk and collect your flowers in a bucket.

**Feverfew**: Before you harvest feverfew, spray the previous night. Early the following morning, harvest the flowers by cutting the stem. Leave just about 4 inches for the flowers to grow for second harvesting.

**Dandelions**: For dandelions, we harvest both leaves and flowers. Depending on the intended use, you can harvest the option that works. To harvest, use a pair of scissors to snip off the flowers. Ensure that you leave sufficient leaves on the stem to allow the flower to continue growing.

**Lavender**: To harvest lavender, you will have to snip the flower with a part of the stem. To ensure that the plant gets a chance to grow again, leave about 4 inches of the stem on the round.

**Ginger**: Ginger is harvested 3 to 4 months after planting. The part that is between the roots, and the stem is the targeted section. The rhizomes of the plant can be cut from the main stem using a knife or any sharp object.

**Garlic**: Harvesting garlic is a simple process. You have to uproot the entire crop from the soil and trim off the roots. After harvesting your garlic, clean it well to remove the soil. Since the herb is usually covered with an outside film, remove it to remain with the clean inner bulb.

**Yarrow**: To harvest yarrow, cut the entire stem halfway. You may pluck it with your hand or use a pair of scissors. If you do not cut well, the flower will not grow. You can harvest yarrow more than twice as long as you cut the stem very well.

**Valerian**: Valerian should be harvested on a warm day. I usually harvest my valerian in spring to get the ideal temperature. The parts that are used include the roots and rhizomes of the plant. To harvest the best roots, wait until they are at least 1 to 2 years old. You should be careful not to dig out the roots as you harvest.

**Thyme**: Thyme is harvested during summer or spring. To harvest, cut the top 5 or 6 inches of the crop. Leave the woody stem to continue growing for future harvesting. Thyme can be harvested throughout the year as long as you cut the sprigs carefully.

**St. John's Wort**: Harvest the buds or the entire stalk once the flowers are in full bloom. The ideal time for harvesting is during summer or spring. You should not harvest flowers that have been sprayed with pesticides.

To harvest, pluck out the buds or cut 2- 3 inches of the stick with the buds.

**Plantain**: For plantain, we can harvest both the leaves and the seed. The seeds should be harvested once they turn brown. Since the herb grows freely and is highly invasive, you should harvest without fear. Harvest the leaves throughout the season.

**Mullein**: For mullein, we harvest the leaves since they carry potent medicinal components. The leaves grow as big as 3 to 6 inches. To harvest, pick the leaves during mid-morning hours. You have to let the morning dew dry out before picking the leaves. Make sure you rinse the leaves well after picking. Do not pick leaves that have been sprayed with pesticides.

**Marshmallow Root**: The roots of this herb are usually harvested in the late fall. Harvest after the plant has dried but right before the ground freezes. Marshmallow should be harvested using a spade to avoid spoiling the roots.

**Oregano**: Harvesting oregano is more like pruning. To harvest the plant, cut it right above two leaves. Retain about 4 inches of the herb in the ground to provide room for further germination.

The harvesting procedures for most of the herbs are the same. For those that need plucking of leaves or trimming the sprig, just use a pair of scissors or cut them directly.

## KEEPING THE GARDEN THRIVING

Planting your herbs is one thing while maintaining a thriving garden is a different story. After planting your herbs, you need to employ regular maintenance techniques that will help your garden flourish. There are some simple steps you can take to ensure that your garden remains thriving throughout the year.

### CHANGE YOUR WATERING SCHEDULE WITH SEASONS

One of the important aspects of herbal gardening is the watering schedule. If you get the water schedule right, your herbs will thrive even without the need to apply fertilizers. The mistake that most herbal gardeners make is to stick to one watering schedule throughout the year. The water needs of most plants change as the year progresses. You should not expect your herbs to use the same amount of water in winter as they use in summer. During the colder months, you should cut watering your herbs by 50 to 70 percent. If you are used to watering your herbs once per week for hotter days, change the schedule to once every 2 weeks in hotter months. The idea is to help your herbs utilize the available water before adding more water to the planters.

Furthermore, you should also consider the location of the plants when watering. There are those who keep their herbs indoors during the cold months. If you happen to move your herbs indoors, you should always water according to the rate of water consumption. Do not add water to the planters before the available one is well-drained.

## KEEP THE WATER IN THE SOIL WITH MULCH

During summers, water might easily evaporate from the soil due to the hot sun. In such seasons, you need to find ways of retaining water in the soil. We have highlighted the water needs of each crop in the sections above. If you are going to provide the ideal water for your crops in summer, you should find ways of retaining it. One of the best water retention methods is to cover the soil with mulch. Use grass and other waste to cover the beds or the planters before watering the plants. Such waste materials will help the soil hold water much longer. It is particularly necessary to use mulch on crops that thrive in sandy soil. Sandy soils drain water very fast and may leave the crop thirsty if you do not retain some in the mulch.

## KEEP WEEDS DOWN IN THE GARDEN

The best way to take care of your garden is by reducing the number of weeds. If you want your herbs to thrive, ensure that weeds are not allowed to grow. It is often not an easy task to keep the weeds out. To ensure that there are no weeds in your beds and planters, thoroughly prepare the soil before growing. You should start by turning the soil several times and let it dry well before planting. If you let the soil dry well, any weed seeds within may die before they start germinating.

Once you plant, stay close to monitor the germination process. Use your hands to pick out any weed that may crop during the first few days. Pay close attention to your crops and weed the garden once every 2 weeks to completely keep the weeds away. If the weeds grow tall beyond your control, plow through the garden and use pesticides to control them. However, I will discourage the use of pesticides on herbal gardens. You should try as much as possible to contain the weeds through other methods, as highlighted above.

## DEAL WITH PESTS

The other way of ensuring that your garden thrives is getting rid of pests. Besides weeds, pests also affect the garden. If pests infest the garden, all your herbs may die or get stranded. To deal with pests, follow the steps provided in the pest control section above. We mainly use natural means of pest control such as weeding, keeping predator animals, and using natural remedies such as ash. However, if the pests get to unbearable levels, you might be forced to use some pesticides. Again, you should only use pesticides on herbal gardens as a measure of last resort. After using pesticides, give your gardens sufficient time for the pesticide to wash away before harvesting.

## FEED YOUR GARDEN

The other way to keep your garden thriving is by providing food for your crops. Each herb has special nutritional needs. In the sections above, we have looked at the nutritional needs of all the herbs we planted. The herbs that have a high requirement for fertilizer should be supplied with fertilizers several times in a year. When providing the fertilizer, you should choose the ideal option for your herb. For instance, we established that Marshmallow demands high phosphorus fertilizers while cayenne pepper requires calcium rich fertilizers. We have provided the soil requirement guide for all the herbs in this book. Look at the guide to help you determine the ideal fertilizer for your crop. For a crop that thrives in alkaline soil, you should use alkaline fertilizers. However, make sure you have the soil tested for pH before you start applying the required fertilizers.

Besides the application of industrial fertilizers, you may prepare natural fertilizers at home. If you are keeping some birds such as chickens at home, they may provide the best manure for your gardens. Simply collect the chicken poop, mix it with some hay and decompose for about 4 months. Use the manure to fertilize your herbs.

## HARVEST REGULARLY

Lastly, you have to harvest your crops regularly for them to thrive. Harvesting gives the crop room to produce fresh branches. Harvesting is similar to pruning in most cases. When you prune your crops, you provide room for the stem to give birth to more branches. For crops that can be harvested and still germinate like the flowers, you should harvest in advance. We have highlighted the ideal harvesting season for each of the flowers. Pick the flowers at the right time to give them an opportunity to flourish for the next season.

## DEALING WITH CHANGING SEASONS

One of the biggest challenges that most gardeners have to deal with is changes in seasons. When transiting from one extreme to another, the crops have to strain to survive. It is your duty to help the crops transit smoothly. There are some steps you can take to deal with season changes. Some of the actions you can taker include:

## KNOW YOUR CLIMATE ZONE

Planting herbs without knowing your climate zone is a ticket for failure. There are some herbs that will not survive in a certain climate, no matter what you do. If you want to survive the harsh season changes experienced in most places across the US, you have to know your zone. We have provided a full guide on choosing the climatic zone. Look at the hardiness zones in the map and choose the crops that do well within your zone. Essentially, some crops are perennial in almost all climate zones. Examine the performance of all the herbs and the zones in which they are perennial. If any of the herbs on our list does not fall within your growing zone, avoid them entirely. If you choose crops that are suitable for your climate zone, you will never have to worry about changes in seasons. A crop that is ideal for all hardiness zones will do well in winter, spring, and summer.

## TIME THE HARVEST

The other way of dealing with season changes is to time your planting and harvesting. With the right timing, you will never have to deal with harsh climatic conditions. For instance, garlic takes about 9 months to mature. If you plant your garlic between September and November, you might just harvest your garlic in time before winter. However, if you wait until January to plant your garlic, you may be forced to wait until winter is over to harvest garlic. Unfortunately, garlic does not fare well under the cold weather. It is, therefore, necessary to get the timing of your season right. If you plant and harvest at the ideal time, you will never have to deal with the harsh temperature changes. For crops that can mature and be harvested in 6 to 9 months, you should be able to deal with them without worrying about season changes.

## KEEP THE SOIL HEALTHY

The other way of dealing with season changes is to ensure that the crops are well fertilized. Most people tend to forget that the crops need fertilizers during winter. Just before the ground starts freezing, ensure that you provide sufficient fertilizer for your crops to take them through the cold season. Ensure that you also provide sufficient water to the soil.

# Chapter 4: Using the Plants and Herbs for Medicinal Purposes

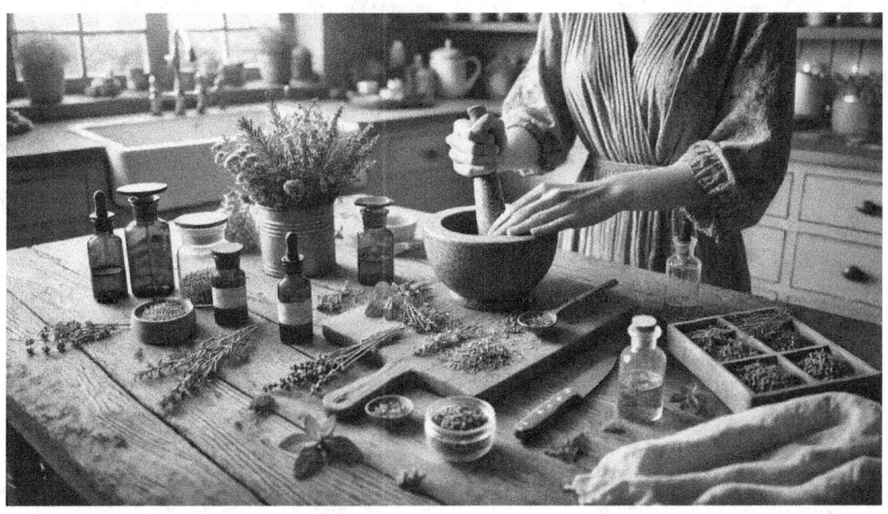

Now that we have looked at the ways to cultivate various herbs, I want us to move the ways of using the herbs. After cultivating and harvesting your herbs, you should use them to treat various conditions. For some of the herbs on this list, we will be using them as part of our daily nutrition, while others will be used to prepare herbal medication. In this chapter, we look at ways to use herbs, including recipes for preparing herbal applications and the ways of using the applications.

There are many ways to use herbal remedies. The herbs that are used to treat internal conditions are mostly ingested, while those that treat external conditions are applied externally. For the purpose of this book, we will mainly focus on the ways of ingesting herbal products. After harvesting the herbs, you need to prepare them into the final form for application.

## BREWING HERBAL TEAS

Herbal teas are the most popular method of ingesting herbs. Since herbal teas are easy to prepare, they are popular among herbal product users. Herbal teas are usually prepared in a similar way to common tea with few exceptions. For instance, herbal tea may be brewed without the addition of sugar, or it might be brewed much longer than regular tea. For any herbal tea to be effective, it must be brewed to the ideal temperature for the medicinal components of the herb to steepen in the water. Most medicinal components can be extracted by boiling the herbs in hot water. In some instances, complex solvents are used to dissolve the herbs in the water. In either way, herbal teas are ideal for all people who prefer taking the herbs in hot beverages.

## HERBAL TINCTURES

The other way of ingesting herbs is by preparing tinctures. Tinctures are the much stronger version of any herbal application. With tinctures, the herb is dissolved in alcohol so that the medicinal components can be concentrated in just a small amount of the tincture. Tinctures are usually very strong and should be prescribed in the right way to avoid serious side effects. Most tinctures are prepared by dissolving the herb in alcohol, although other solvent methods can be used. In most cases, alcohol is used to dissolve herbs that do not respond to water-based solvents.

## EATING LEAVES AND ROOTS

The other option when it comes to ingesting herbs is to eat the leaves or roots. Many medicinal herbs can be eaten directly without the need to brew or prepare tinctures. Some herbs such as rosemary, thyme, coriander, and parsley can be eaten raw. Leaves are easy to eat raw since they are much tender as compared to roots and the stalk. However, some people eat raw roots and stalks without a problem.

While a person can eat raw herbs, some are usually very bitter. Most herbs are bitter if consumed raw. For this reason, people avoid eating raw leaves and roots. The best way of consuming raw leaves and roots is by combining them with other vegetables in salads or making them part of your diet. For instance, you could chop a few rosemary leaves in your salad and season with cayenne pepper. The salad will not have the bitterness presented in eating raw herbs.

There are many ways you could prepare the herbs we planted above to cure various conditions. Each of the herbs has different applications from the other. I am going to help you prepare the teas and tinctures for each of these herbs and also show you ways you could serve them raw in foods to treat certain conditions.

Basil can be used to treat conditions such as loss of appetite, intestinal gas, warts, and kidney conditions, among others. If you suffer from any of these conditions, you can take basil tea either as a treatment or on a regular basis. For those suffering from kidney conditions, drink basil tea instead of regular tea.

## BASIL TEA

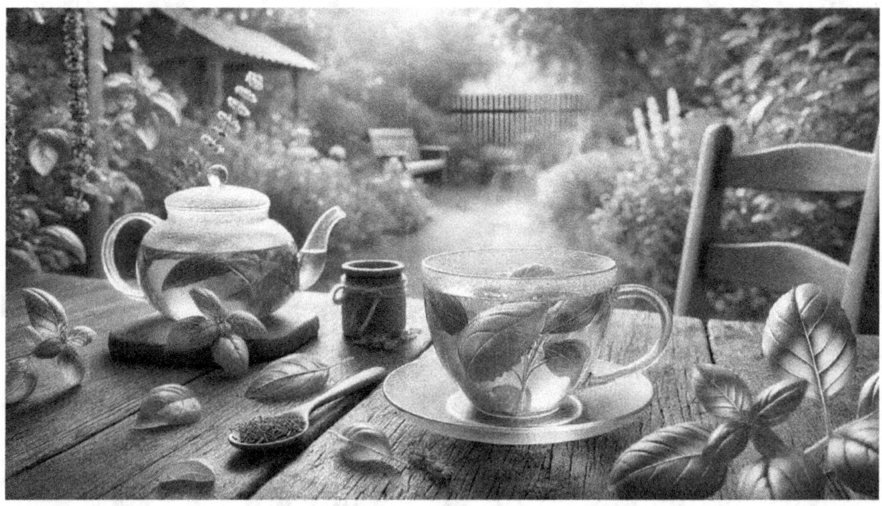

This tea is for 2 people, each drinking 1 cup of tea.

1/2 cup of basil leaves

2.5 cups of water

2 teaspoons of tea leaves

1 teaspoon of sugar or 2 teaspoons of honey

1 cup of milk

1. In a small kettle, bring the water and basil leaves to a boil.

2. Once that boils, lower the heat and allow the tea to brew for about 5 more minutes.

3. Now add the leaves and sugar/honey as indicated or to your preferred taste.

4. Add the milk and strain the tea into a jug or cups.

This tea should be consumed without milk if you are trying to treat stomach upset.

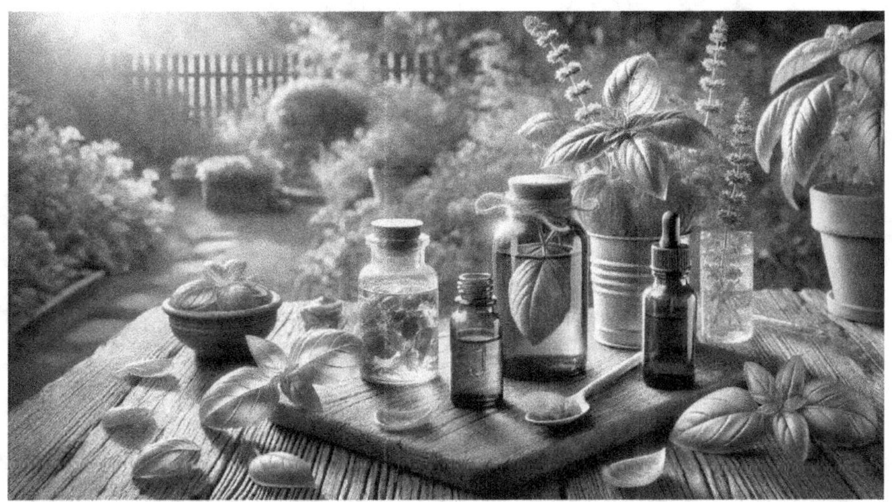

Basil tinctures are powerful and can be taken daily as medicine to treat most conditions that the herb treats.

1-quart size jar with lid

5 cups of clear vodka

1 ounce of basil leaves (fresh or dried)

1. Place the cleaned basil leaves into a clean, sterilized glass jar.

2. Measure out about 3 cups of the vodka and add to the jar with the basil leaves. You may also use vegetable glycerin for this purpose, but your tincture will have a short lifespan.

3. Place the lid on your jar and mix vigorously.

4. Label the jars with the date and ingredients and store them in a cool, dry place such as the kitchen cabinet.

5. Shake your tincture once or twice every week for about 5 weeks.

6. Strain your basil tincture into a different glass jar and refrigerate.

Your basil tincture is ready for consumption. You can take 1 teaspoon per day to treat kidney conditions or warts. If you are not suffering from a specific condition, you could still make it part of your diet by mixing it with salad dressing or vegetable sauce.

For those who wish to make basil part of their daily lifestyle, it is better when used to cook regular foods. You can cook almost any food with basil. The best dish to serve with basil is beef.

2 tablespoons of vegetable oil

2 shallots, thinly sliced

7 sliced garlic cloves (more or less to taste)

1 tablespoon of minced fresh ginger

1/2 thinly sliced red bell pepper

1 lb. ground beef

2 teaspoons of brown sugar

2 tablespoons of fish sauce

6 tablespoons of low sodium soy sauce

3 teaspoons of oyster sauce

2 tablespoons of Asian garlic chili paste

1/2 cup of low sodium beef broth

1/4 cup of tap water

1 teaspoon of cornstarch

1 cup of sliced basil leaves

1. Heat a large skillet over medium heat and add the cooking oil. Allow the oil to cook on medium heat and add the shallots, garlic, ginger, and bell peppers. Fry all the spices and vegetables for about 5 minutes.

2. Keep the vegetables aside and turn the heat to high. Add ground beef to your skillet, breaking it apart with a spoon.

3. In a small bowl, mix the oyster sauce, cornstarch, and beef broth with a little water and add to the pan. Cook the combination for about 2 minutes.

4. Now add the basil to your mixture above and stir fry until wilted.

Serve your basil beef with the vegetables prepared while still hot. This combination can be served with rice or noodles.

## ROSEMARY RECIPES

Rosemary is one of the most beneficial herbs on this list. This herb can be used to treat a variety of conditions, including bronchial asthma, prostate disorders, inflammatory diseases, liver toxicity, improving memory, and preventing cancer, among others. Although rosemary has so many uses, most herbalists use it as a detox product. For this reason, the best way to consume rosemary is through rosemary tea. Brewing rosemary tea daily will help you live a long healthy life with a body free of toxins.

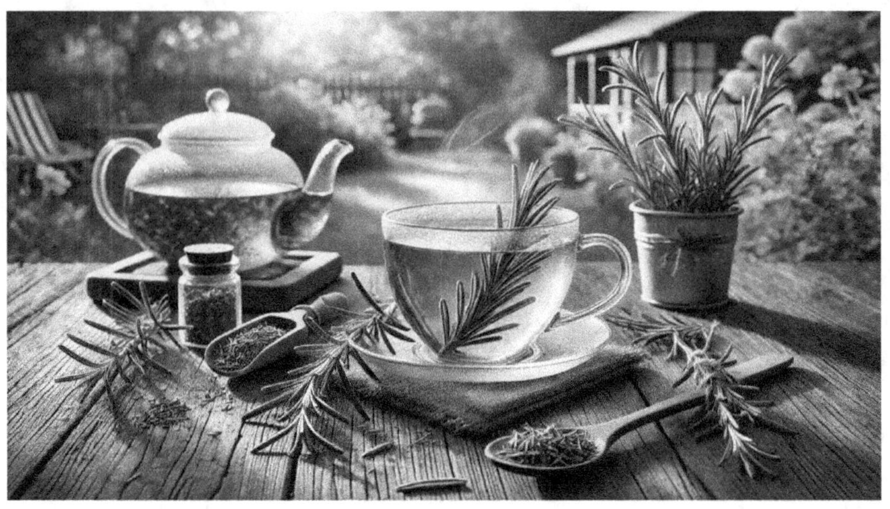

3 teaspoons of rosemary leaves or 1 teaspoon of dried rosemary leaves

2 cups of water

1 teaspoon of sugar or 2 teaspoons of honey

1. Steep the rosemary leaves in water for about 5 minutes or more over medium heat. The longer you steep the leaves, the stronger the tea.

2. Once your tea boils and the herbs steep to your preferred level, remove from heat and drain into a cup.

3. Add the sugar or honey and mix well.

4. Enjoy your tea with your preferred dish.

Note: Rosemary tea might get bitter if you steep for too long. If you are using fresh leaves, just steep for 5 minutes and drink with the leaves inside the cup.

## ROSEMARY TINCTURE

The best rosemary ingestible for all those looking for medical help is the rosemary tincture. Here is a short recipe to make your tincture at home.

1 cup of sliced, fresh rosemary leaves

350 ml bottle of 80 proof vodka.

1. Place the leaves in a glass jar and top up with 2 cups of 80 proof vodka

2. Let the leaves stay in your jar for about 6 weeks; shake daily.

3. After six weeks, drain your tincture into a small bottle and store it in the refrigerator.

Take 1 teaspoon for any of the diseases mentioned above. You may also make this tincture part of your daily diet by combining it with sauces, butter, or salads.

## ROSEMARY GARLIC BEEF ROAST

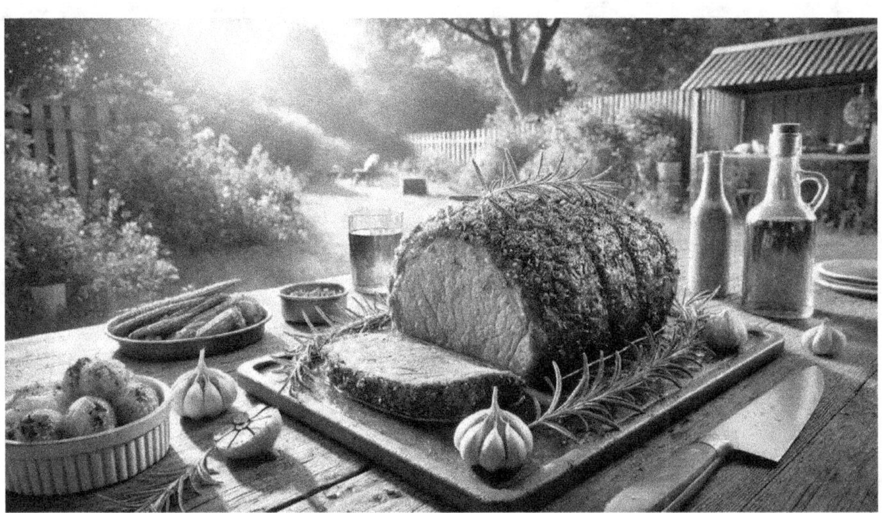

Besides the tea and tincture, you can also use rosemary to prepare a delicious roast.

3 lbs. of boneless rib eye roast

1/4 cup of freshly plucked rosemary, chopped

1/4 cup of garlic, chopped

Freshly ground cayenne pepper

1 teaspoon of salt (more or less to taste)

4 tablespoons of olive oil, divided into 2

4 tablespoons of butter, divided into 2

4 cups of mushrooms sliced

1 cup of stock

1. Preheat the oven to 350 F.

2. Tie the roast and season with salt and pepper

3. Mix the rosemary and garlic together in a small bowl and add about 2 tablespoons of olive oil. Mix well and reserve.

4. In a cast-iron skillet on medium heat, add the remaining 2 tablespoons of olive oil. Cook the oil to smoking hot then sear all the sides of the meat for about 2 minutes per side.

5. Remove the beef from the skillet and brush the herb garlic mixture on both sides. Transfer the roast into the oven and cook for about 1 to 2 hours. Usually, I would just roast the beef in the iron skillet, but you can use a roasting pan.

6. Let the meat cool down to about 70 degrees F before serving.

Bring the skillet to the stovetop. Add the stock to the pan and deglaze. Allow it to simmer until thick, then add the mushrooms to the sauce. Add in the remaining 2 tablespoons of butter and stir until silky.

With that, you have your rosemary garlic beef ready for serving. You should make it part of your lifestyle to cook with herbs such as rosemary and garlic for overall improved health.

# CAYENNE PEPPER RECIPES

Cayenne pepper is one of the common herbs in most homes. It is loved due to its culinary and health benefits. Cayenne is used to season foods alongside other additives. The pepper offers several health benefits, including treating blood circulatory problems, stopping bleeding, and reducing the risk of heart attacks. If you have a family member at the risk of experiencing a heart attack, you should make cayenne part of your daily meals. Here are some easy to prepare recipes that include cayenne pepper.

4 cups of water

1 piece of ginger, peeled and pounded

2 tablespoons of lemon juice

1/2 tablespoon of ground cayenne pepper

Honey/sugar for sweetening

1. Mix the ginger with 3 cups of water in a saucepan.

2. Bring the water to a boil and let it simmer on low heat for about 10 to 15 minutes.

3. Add cayenne pepper to the water and let it continue simmering for another 3 minutes.

Remove the tea from the heat and add the 2 tablespoons of lemon juice. Sweeten the tea with honey or sugar to your desired level.

Besides the tea, an ideal way to ingest cayenne is through a cayenne tincture. Cayenne tinctures can be used as a sauce in most foods and can also be taken directly. Here is a simple recipe for the tincture.

1/2 cup of ground cayenne pepper

350 ml (about 1 ½ cups) of high proof clear vodka or apple cider vinegar

1. Fill a glass jar with vodka to the halfway mark. You may use apple cider vinegar or glycerin for the same purpose.

2. Add the cayenne pepper to your alcohol and tighten the lid.

3. Store the jar in a cool dark place. After 6 weeks, drain the tincture through cheesecloth to remove the pepper.

4. Pour the tincture into a small colored bottle for use.

Cayenne tinctures can be taken daily by individuals who suffer from blood circulation problems. Some of the symptoms of blood circulation include dizziness, low sexual libido, and heart attacks, among others. If you experience such symptoms, use about 1/2 a teaspoon of cayenne tincture every morning.

## CAYENNE PEPPER GRILLED SALMON

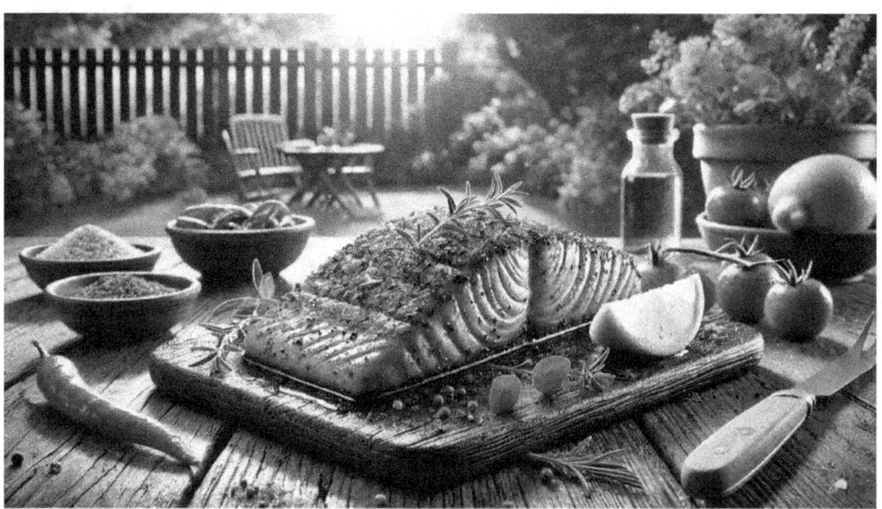

If you are not a fan of tea or tinctures, you have the option of using the pepper for seasoning your grilled beef, chicken, turkey, pork, or fish. Here is a simple recipe for grilled salmon seasoned with cayenne pepper.

2 tablespoons of ground paprika

1 tablespoon of ground cayenne pepper

1 tablespoon of onion powder

2 teaspoons of salt

1/2 teaspoon of ground white pepper

1/2 teaspoon of ground black pepper

1/4 teaspoon of dried thyme

1/4 teaspoon of dried basil

1/4 teaspoon of dried oregano

6 ounces of salmon fillet

1/2 cup of unsalted butter

1. In a small bowl, mix the spices together (paprika, cayenne, onion powder, salt, white pepper, black pepper, thyme, basil, and oregano).

2. Brush the salmon filets with a 1/4 cup of butter on both sides and sprinkle the spices mixture evenly over the filets.

3. Drizzle each fillet on one side with 1/2 the butter.

4. Place a large skillet on high heat and cook the salmon, butter side down, for about 3 minutes or until it is blackened.

5. Turn the fillet, drizzle with the remaining butter, and continue cooking until the other side is blackened.

With that, you have your salmon seasoned with cayenne. If you find this recipe applicable, you should make it a part of your lifestyle.

# ALOE VERA RECIPES

Aloe vera is one of the most popular herbs and can be used to treat many conditions. It is mainly used to treat burns, digestive problems, and acne, among others. Although aloe vera is mostly applied for skin conditions, it can also be used to treat indigestion and other stomach issues.

## ALOE VERA TEA

1 teaspoon of dried and ground aloe vera

I teaspoon of tea leaves of your choice

2 teaspoons of lemon juice

1 liter of freshly boiled water

sliced strawberries

mint leaves

Ice cubes

1. Pour the boiled water over the ground aloe vera and the tea leaves in a heatproof jug.

2. Allow the tea to brew for about 10 minutes before adding the lemon juice.

3. Remove the tea from heat and decant to remove the tea and aloe vera leaves.

Allow your tea to cool completely. You may place it in the refrigerator to speed up the cooling process. Once the tea is cool, fill a glass to the 3/4 mark with ice cubes and pour the tea over them. Garnish with strawberry slices and fresh mint.

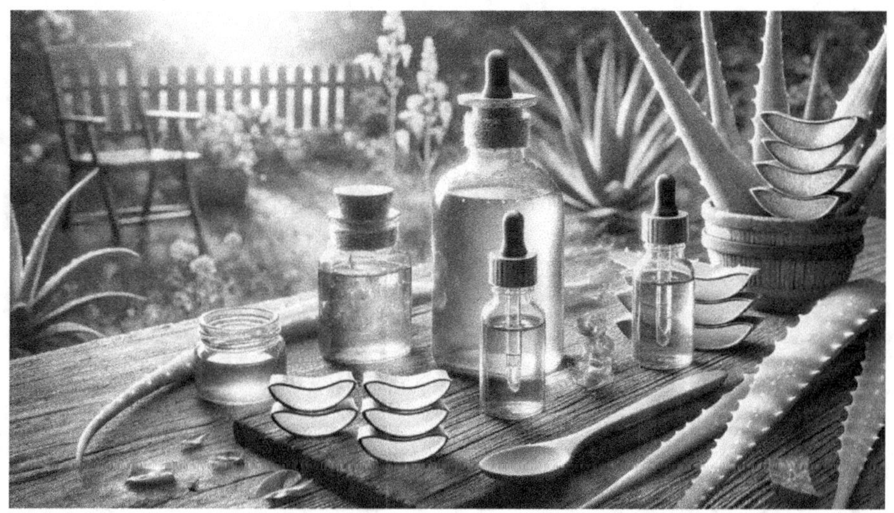

Aloe vera tinctures are the ideal application for those who cannot bear drinking the bitter tea. Since aloe vera is a very bitter herb, the tea prepared is very bitter too. Although tinctures are also bitter, you do not have to take large amounts. You may be required to drink about a full glass of aloe vera tea each day; however, you may only have to take a single teaspoon of the tincture for the same health benefits. Here is a simple step by step process of preparing aloe vera tinctures.

1 full aloe vera leaf

55 ml of 96 proof medicinal alcohol

45 ml distilled water

1. Cut the tip of the aloe vera leaf from about 2 centimeters from the base along with the spines and discard.

2. Cut the remaining fleshy part of the leaf into 3 sections and blend until it turns into a homogeneous semi-liquid paste.

4. Now add the distilled water and the alcohol to the liquid aloe vera and mix well with the blender until homogeneous.

5. Put the liquid aloe vera and alcohol mixture in a bottle and let it stay in a cool dark place for about 20 days. After 20 days, open the bottle and filter using cheesecloth into bottles.

For a longer lifespan, refrigerate.

The base tincture can be used for many purposes. You can use it to prepare herbal tea, make infusions, tonics, and prepare skin applications such as creams and salves.

## ALOE VERA SMOOTHIE

Since aloe vera is not ideal for cooked or grilled foods, we will prepare a simple aloe vera smoothie. The fresh smoothie provides an easy option for drinking aloe vera for those who are afraid of the bitter taste.

1 tablespoon aloe vera tincture according to the recipe above

1 banana

1/2 cup of strawberries

1/4 cup ice

1 1/2 cup of coconut milk

1. Place all the ingredients in a blender and blend at high speed for about 2 to 3 minutes until it forms smooth peaks.

2. Taste the smoothie and add coconut milk to taste until it attains your desired thickness.

3. Add the smoothie to a glass and top with fresh fruit or shredded coconut.

Enjoy your smoothie immediately or refrigerate for 24 hours.

## BURDOCK RECIPES

Burdock roots are known to offer diverse health benefits, including the ability to reduce bacterial infection, improve urine flow, reduce fevers, and treat colds.

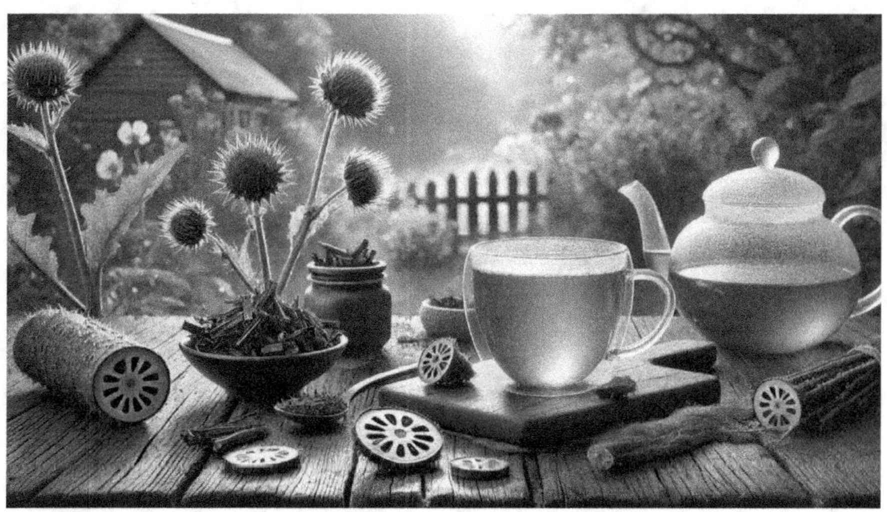

1 teaspoon of burdock root

1 teaspoon of dried dandelion root

2 dried red clover flowers

Dried peppermint leaves to taste

1. Combine all the ingredients and place them into a large mug.

2. Add boiling water to the ingredients and allow it steep for about 30 minutes.

3. Strain the mixture to enjoy your tea.

Burdock tea is very healthy and offers the best option for those who wish to tap into the health benefits of the burdock herb. The tea can help stimulate the kidney and can also be applied externally to treat acne and eczema.

## BURDOCK TINCTURE

For those who are not in a position to make tea or those who find the taste unbearable, the other option is to prepare a burdock root tincture. The tincture can be used in cooking and can also be served with most foods. Here is a simple recipe for burdock root tincture.

1 medium-sized burdock root

50 ml of 80 percent proof vodka

1. Chop the root into small pieces and fill a Mason jar to the halfway mark.

2. Cover the chopped roots with the 80 proof vodka to within 1 inch of the top.

3. Let the tincture infuse in a cool dark place for about 1 month. Shake the jar regularly to expedite the process.

4. After a month, strain the tincture through a fine sieve or cheesecloth and store it in the refrigerator.

## GRILLED BEEF WITH BURDOCK ROOT

Teas and tinctures may taste unbearable for most herbal users. The best solution then becomes finding a way of serving the herbs with tasty grilled foods. Burdock roots can be used in grilling beef, chicken, or fish. Here is a simple recipe for grilled beef.

About ½ lb. of beef shoulder offcuts

¾ cup of burdock roots

1 knob of ginger

1 tablespoon of cooking sake

2 tablespoons of hon-mirin

1 tablespoon of brown sugar

1 teaspoon of soy sauce

1/4 teaspoon of salt

1 tablespoon of vegetable oil

1 sansho leaf

1. Scrub the bark of the burdock root clean and chop the root into small pieces. Soak the root in water for about 3 minutes then drain the water off.

2. Heat some oil in a frying pan and sauté the shoulder cut until brown.

3. Once it browns, add the julienned ginger and turn the heat to low.

4. Add the condiments to your beef in the listed order and stir. Add burdock root and continue mixing.

5. Pour enough water into the pan to soak the ingredients and simmer on medium heat.

Serve with pounded sansho leaves.

With that, you have a mouthwatering dish of grilled beef with burdock roots. The beneficial compounds in the roots are infused into the steak, providing you with a tasty and healthy dish for the entire family.

## GOLDENSEAL RECIPES

Although goldenseal is not a common herb in most homes, it should be. Goldenseal has plenty of health benefits that can be tapped by making it part of a daily diet. The herb can be used to treat digestive disorders, stomach pain, peptic ulcers, diarrhea, and common colds. Here are a few goldenseal recipes that may help you treat some of these conditions.

## GOLDENSEAL TEA

1 teaspoon of dried and pounded goldenseal root/leaves

2 cups of boiling water

1 teaspoon of lemon juice

1 teaspoon of honey or sugar

1. While the water boils in a kettle, place 1 teaspoon of goldenseal powder into a cup.

2. Pour the steaming hot water over the herbs and allow too steep for about 10 minutes.

3. Strain the tea to a different cup and serve while hot.

To improve the taste, add the lemon juice and a teaspoon of honey and mix well.

Note: The tea might have a bitter taste, and most people are unable to tolerate it. However, adding a bit of honey and lemon helps reduce the bitterness. If you feel that the tea is too bitter, try adding a bit more honey. This recipe is ideal for those who wish to use goldenseal to treat common colds.

## GOLDENSEAL TINCTURE

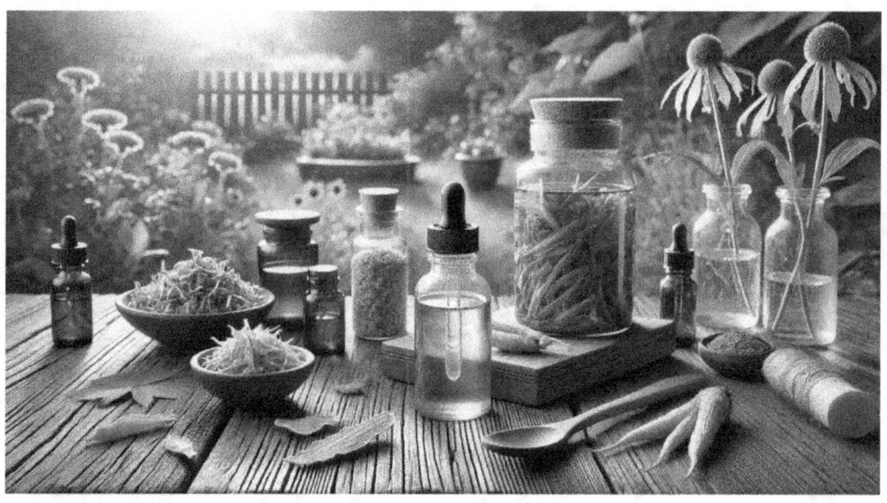

Besides goldenseal tea, you may use a goldenseal tincture to treat any of the above conditions. The tincture works particularly well for those who suffer from peptic ulcers and those who have digestive problems. Taking a teaspoon of the tincture will completely alleviate any digestive problem. Here is a recipe for the tincture.

1 cup of finely chopped goldenseal leaves or 1/2 a cup of chopped roots

½ to 1 cup (or a little more) of high proof vodka

1. Place the chopped herbs in a glass jar and label it with the current date and name of the herbs.

2. Add enough vodka to completely cover the herbs.

3. Cover the glass jar with a tightly fitting lid and place in a cool dark room for about 2 to 3 weeks.

4. Shake your tincture 2 to 3 times every week until ready.

5. After 3 weeks, strain your tincture through cheesecloth into a different glass jar.

6. Allow your tincture to settle in a glass jar overnight before filtering a second time through a filter paper.

Store in a small colored tincture bottle with labels. Make sure your final tincture does not become exposed to direct sunlight.

## CALENDULA RECIPES

Calendula is an herb that can be used to treat a variety of conditions and also used in various foods. For treating specific conditions, calendula can be brewed in teas and served in some foods. The herb is used to treat menstrual cramps, sore throats, reduce fever, prevent muscle spasms, and prevent cancer.

## CALENDULA TEA

1 cup of water

1 teaspoon of calendula flowers

1. Gently pull apart the petals of the flower and place them in a dehydrator.

2. Set the dehydrator to 90 degrees F for 12 hours.

3. After 12 hours, pull the flowers out and rub them in your palms to feel any moisture. If they are not dried, continue dehydrating for up to 3 more hours.

4. Once the flowers are fully dehydrated, store them in a Mason jar until they are ready for brewing tea.

5. To brew tea, bring about 2 cups of water to a boil.

6. Add about one tablespoon of the dried petals to a cup and top it up with water. Allow it too steep for about 10 to 12 minutes.

Drink your tea while it's still hot. You may add a sweetener such as honey or sugar.

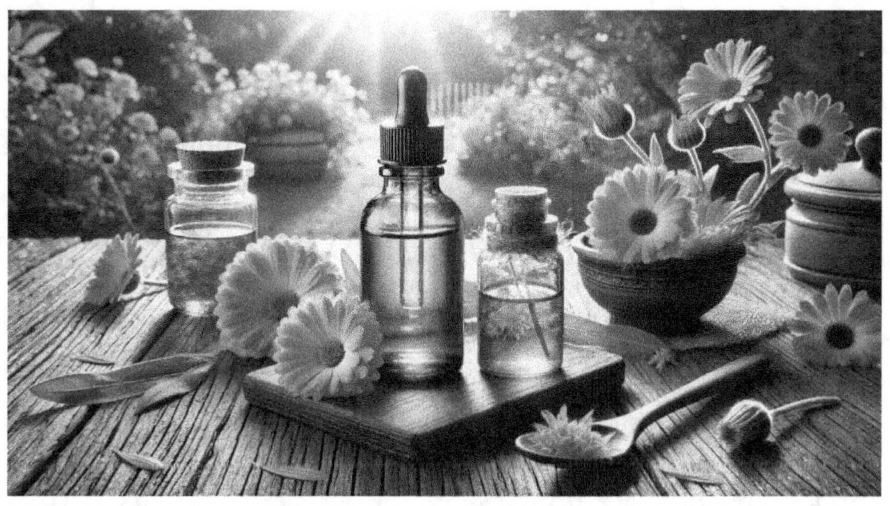

A calendula tincture can be used to treat all the conditions, as mentioned above, more effectively than tea. Here's a simple recipe for the tincture.

1/4 cup of calendula petals, finely chopped

200 ml (about 1 cup) of clear vodka, 80 proof or above

1. Place the finely chopped calendula petals into a Mason jar to the halfway mark.

2. Top up the jar with vodka to within 1 inch of full. Place on a lid and tighten well.

3. Store your tincture in a cool dark place for about 4 weeks for the flowers to infuse into the alcohol.

4. After 4 weeks, filter the tincture through a fine sieve or cheesecloth into a clean Mason jar.

5. After transferring to the jar, let the tincture settle in the jar for about 12 hours.

6. Using filter papers, filter the tincture into colored glass bottles for storage.

Store your calendula tincture in a cool dark place for use for about 6 months.

The tincture prepared in this recipe can be used to prepare external applications but can also be ingested. If you are using calendula to treat indigestion, this product is the ideal option. Just use 1 teaspoon of the tincture each day to treat ulcers or prevent cancer.

Finally, if you do not enjoy the bitter taste associated with calendula, you have the option of cooking with calendula. This herb does not work well on grilled foods such as meat but can be used to prepare special dishes such as this Spanish paella. Here is the recipe.

3 cups of chicken broth

2 cups of uncooked long-grain rice

1 cup of chopped onions

4 cloves of garlic, minced and divided

1 teaspoon of salt

1/2 teaspoon of turmeric

1/4 teaspoon of cayenne pepper

1 bay leaf

1 green pepper, julienned

3 sliced green onions

1 teaspoon of minced parsley

1 teaspoon of dried thyme

1/4 teaspoon of hot pepper sauce

2 tablespoons of olive oil

1 cup of fresh mushroom, sliced

2 medium-sized tomatoes

1 package of frozen peas

1/2 pounds of fresh frozen uncooked shrimp

1 pound of boneless chicken breasts, sliced

2 tablespoons of lemon juice

1/2 cup of calendula petals

1. In a medium-sized saucepan, combine the onions, rice, half the garlic, salt, turmeric, pepper, and bay leaf.

2. Bring the above ingredients to a boil over medium heat, then reduce to low heat and simmer for about 20 minutes.

3. While the rice softens, sauté the green pepper, onions, parsley, garlic, thyme, hot, and pepper sauce in oil for about 2 minutes.

4. Add mushrooms to your spices and cook until the green peppers turn tender.

5. Add the tomato and peas and heat through. Discard the bay leaf and add rice mixture to the vegetable mixture and keep warm over medium heat.

6. In a different skillet, cook the shrimp in lemon juice for 2 minutes and add the chicken. Cook until the chicken turns brown and the shrimp is fully cooked.

7. Now add the rice and the vegetables with calendula. Toss and serve immediately.

With this recipe, you will have prepared tasty Spanish paella that can be served for dinner or lunch. If you enjoy chicken with rice, you could use this recipe to make your meal healthier. This recipe is for those who prefer enjoying herbs in foods rather than those who wish to use it for direct treatment of a certain condition.

## CHICKWEED RECIPES

Chickweed is not a commonly used herb, but it has plenty of health benefits. This herb can be used to treat inflammatory conditions, fighting germs, and promoting weight loss. Here are a few recipes that can help you enjoy chickweed as part of your daily diet.

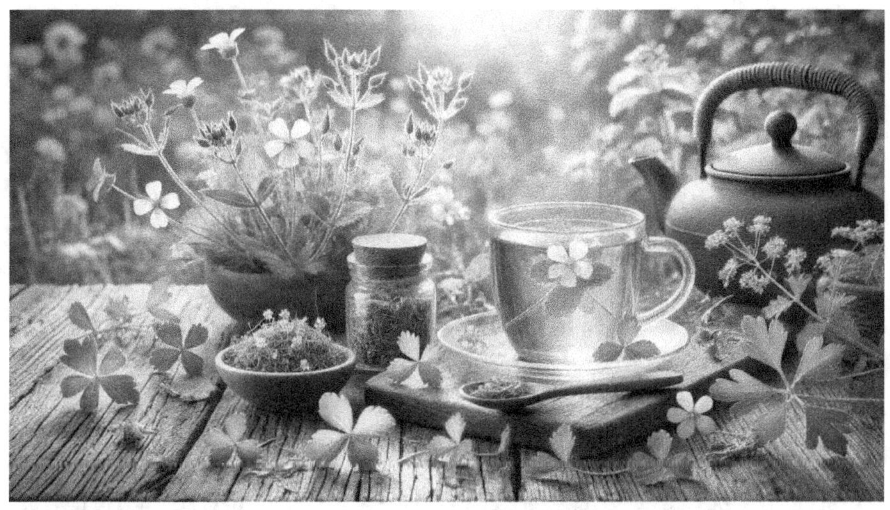

Chickweed tea is somewhat bitter and should only be prepared by those who are willing to persevere the bitterness.

1 cup dried chickweed leaves

3 cups of water

2 tablespoons of lemon juice

1 tablespoon of honey

1. To make your chickweed tea, add 1 cup of the dried chickweed leaves to 3 cups of boiling water and simmer over medium heat for 5 minutes.

2. Filter out the leaves and prepare a cup of tea by mixing with lemon and honey.

3. Drink about 1 cup of chickweed tea every 3 hours to enhance your results if you are trying to lose weight.

With this recipe, you can improve your appetite, burn fat, and treat internal inflammatory conditions.

## CHICKWEED TINCTURE

Chickweed tincture is the best option for those who wish to apply it externally. It can also be used to prepare teas and other food additives such as sauce. Here is a simple recipe for your chickweed tincture.

1 cup of good quality vodka

3/4 cup of fresh chickweed

Sterilized Mason jar

1. Gather fresh chickweed in the morning when it is free of all moisture.

2. Chop your herb finely and place it into a Mason jar.

3. Pour vodka over the chickweed until all the leaves are fully submerged.

4. Place a lid on the jar and tighten well.

5. Let the tincture sit under direct sunlight for about 4 to 8 weeks. Shake the bottle every couple of weeks to agitate the infusion process.

6. After 8 weeks, strain through a fine sieve or cheesecloth.

Store your chickweed tincture in a cool dark place for use for 1 year or more.

Chamomile is one of the most popular herbs when it comes to culinary uses. This herb is not only loved due to its spicing ability but also due to its health benefits. Some of the health benefits of chamomile include treatment of hay fever, muscle spasms, menstrual disorders, rheumatoid, ulcers, and insomnia, among others.

## CHAMOMILE TEA

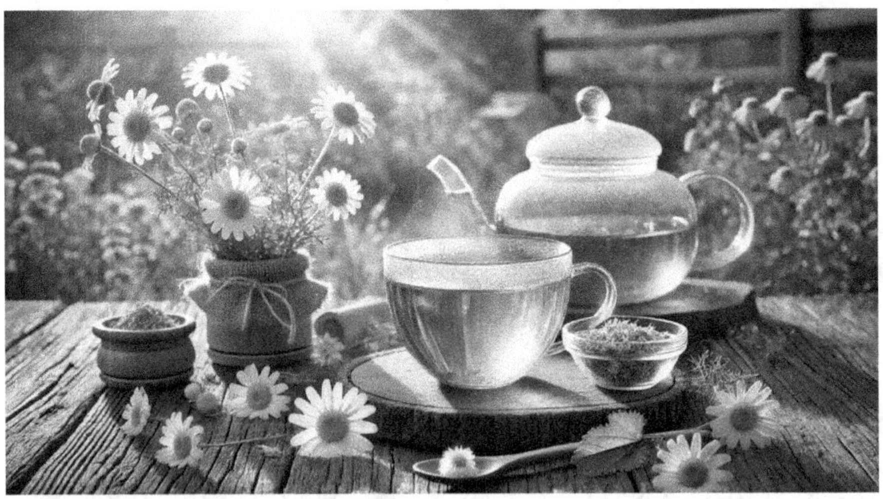

Chamomile tea is among the most popular types of tea and is often used to treat fever and muscle spasms.

2 cups of water

1/4 cup of chamomile powder

1 cup of cold whole milk

1 tablespoon of honey

1 spoon of ground cinnamon

1. Bring water to a boil in a small saucepan.

2. Add the chamomile to the water and let it simmer for about 5 minutes.

3. Filter the tea into a cup and cover it with plastic wrap.

4. While the tea is resting, heat milk in a small saucepan while whisking until it is warm and frothy.

5. Once it is ready, mix about a 1/4 cup of milk with 3/4 cup of the tea prepared earlier.

6. Add the honey and mix well.

7. Top the cup of tea with some milk froth and sprinkle cinnamon powder on top.

Enjoy your chamomile tea at any time of the day.

## CHAMOMILE TINCTURES

The other option is to prepare a chamomile tincture instead of taking the tea. Here is a quick chamomile tincture recipe.

1 cup of dried chamomile flowers

2 cups of boiling water

2 cups of 90 proof vodka

Quart-size glass jars with airtight lids

1. Put the fresh chopped flowers in a quart-size jar and pour boiling water on top to just cover them.

2. Pour vodka on top to fill the Mason jar and tightly cover the jar with a lid.

3. Store the tincture in a cool dark place and store for about 6 weeks to infuse. Shake at least once every week to agitate the process.

4. After 6 weeks, remove from the cabinet and strain through a cheesecloth.

Store the tincture in a clear glass bottle or jar.

## CHAMOMILE TOAST CRUNCH

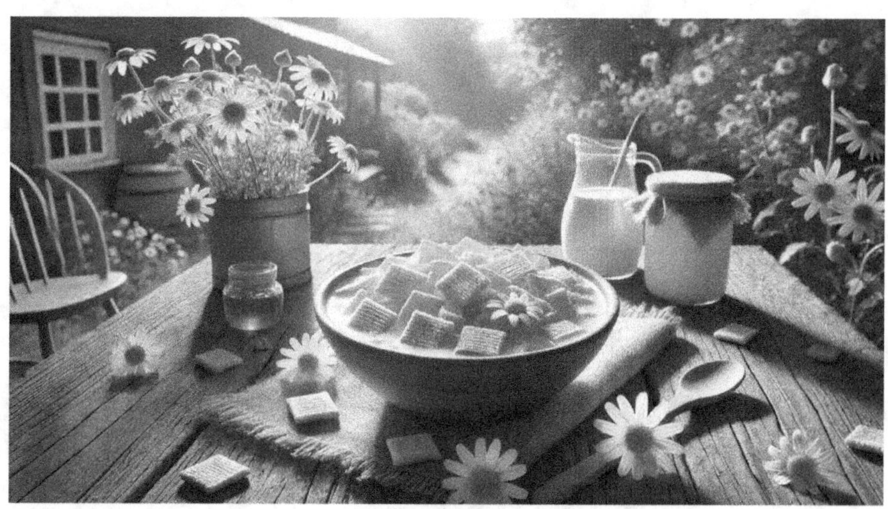

The other option is to prepare your food with chamomile. You can prepare toast with chamomile for a healthy breakfast. Here is the recipe.

1 cup of half-and-half

1/4 cup of dried chamomile

1 can of sweetened condensed milk

1 stick unsalted butter

4 thick slices of bakery bread

Sugar

1. Warm the half-and-half to almost a simmer, then turn off the heat and add the chamomile.

2. Steep while covered for about 10 minutes.

3. Add condensed milk.

4. Spread 2 tablespoons of softened butter on each slice of bread.

5. Toast the bread until it is slightly browned.

6. Dip each of the toast in sugar and sprinkle on a bit more to coat

7. Now torch the sugared toast on a metal rack over a pan. Hold the torch nozzle 3 inches from your toast and move it across the surface of the slices. Tip your pan to aim the melted sugar towards the un-melted sugar section.

Serve your chamomile toast crunch while warm.

With that, you have your chamomile toast ready. Serve the bread in a heavy puddle of sweet chamomile milk.

# FEVERFEW RECIPES

The most popular use of feverfew is reducing fevers. This explains its name. However, this herb has many other uses, including treating stomach ache, rheumatoid arthritis, reduced labor pain during childbirth, insect bites, and infertility, among other uses. Here are some quick feverfew recipes you can prepare.

## FEVERFEW TEA

1/4 cup of feverfew leaves or blooms

1 cup of boiling water

1 tablespoon of lemon juice

1 tablespoon of honey

1. Add the fresh blooms or leaves to a cup of boiling water and allow them too steep for about 5 minutes.

2. After 5 minutes, strain the tea into a cup and cool for 10 minutes.

3. Add the lemon juice and honey and stir well.

Enjoy your feverfew tea.

Fever few tea is mainly used to treat fevers and migraines. However, you may also make a cup of feverfew tea every morning if you suffer from arthritis and rheumatism.

## FEVERFEW TINCTURES

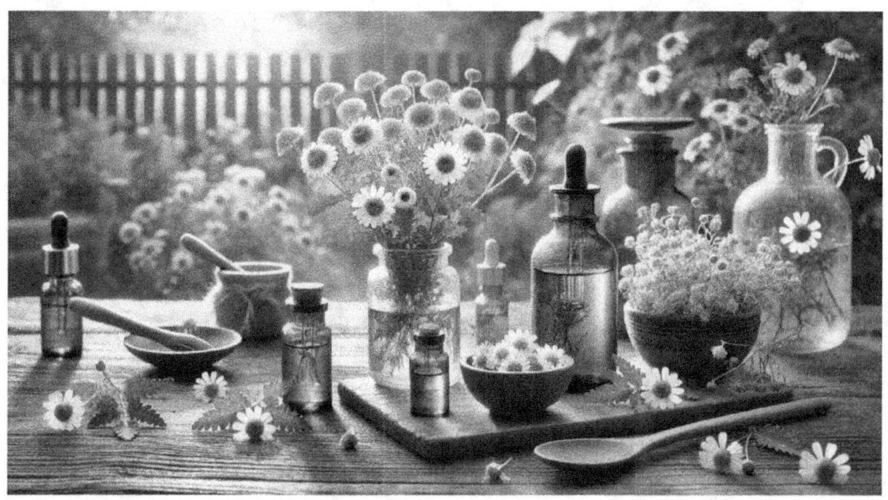

Besides treating headaches and fever, this herb can also be used as an anti-inflammatory to reduce pain associated with arthritis. The best way of using feverfew to treat arthritis is by preparing a tincture. The feverfew tincture can be combined with gels and oils to be applied as salves externally. Here is the recipe.

1 cup of chopped, fresh feverfew flowers

1 cup of clear, high proof vodka

1. Soak the chopped flowers in the vodka in a Mason jar and cap with a tight lid.

2. Keep the tincture in a cool dark place for about 4 weeks, then filter with a cheesecloth.

3. Store the tincture in a colored bottle until time for use.

Since the tincture is made with alcohol, it has a lifespan of up to 3 years. However, if you use glycerin to infuse the herbs, you should use your tincture in less than a year.

The tinctures prepared here can be used to treat arthritis pain when applied externally.

## DANDELION RECIPES

Dandelions are popular flowers and are used to treat a variety of diseases. Some of the diseases that dandelions treat include blood pressure, blood sugar, and high cholesterol. Here are a few recipes you may use to prepare dandelion ingestible.

## DANDELION TEA

Dandelion tea is easy to prepare and offers a refreshing, sweet taste. If you are a fan of tea, you will find this healthy and enticing.

1 ounce of fresh dandelion flowers

1 cup of hot water

2 to 3 tablespoons of dried stevia leaf

1/2 cups of dried raspberry leaf

3 ounces of cold water

The juice of 3 limes

1. Place your freshly picked dandelions into a colander and separate the yellow parts from the leaves. Discard the leaves and the stalk.

2. Rinse the dandelions in flowing water and put them in a jar.

3. Pour hot water over the dandelions such that they are just submerged and steep for 5 minutes.

4. In a separate jar, pour some hot water over stevia or raspberry leaves and steep for 5 minutes.

5. Strain the sweetened water into the jar with dandelions and mix well.

6. Strain the dandelion tea into a different jar and sweeten with sugar, honey, or lemon.

7. Refrigerate your tea for about 4 hours or until it is completely chilled.

8. Use the tea within 36 hours of preparation.

## DANDELION TINCTURE

The dandelion tincture is easy to prepare and is less bitter as compared to the tea. This tincture can be used for various purposes, including internal and external applications.

1 cup of chopped dandelion, mix roots, leaves, and flowers

50 ml of vodka

1. Wash the chopped dandelions with plenty of water to remove any dirt.

2. Place the dandelions in a glass jar and fill it with 100 proof vodka.

3. Use a chopstick to poke around to ensure that all the dandelions are submerged.

4. Place the lid and tighten to ensure that it is airtight.

5. Store in a cool, dry place for about 6 weeks.

6. Shake the jar 2 -3 times every week to accelerate the infusion process.

7. Once the tincture is ready, strain out the plant materials and dispose of it.

8. Pour the tincture into a clean colored bottle and store in a cool dark place. You can use this tincture for about 2 to 3 years without a problem.

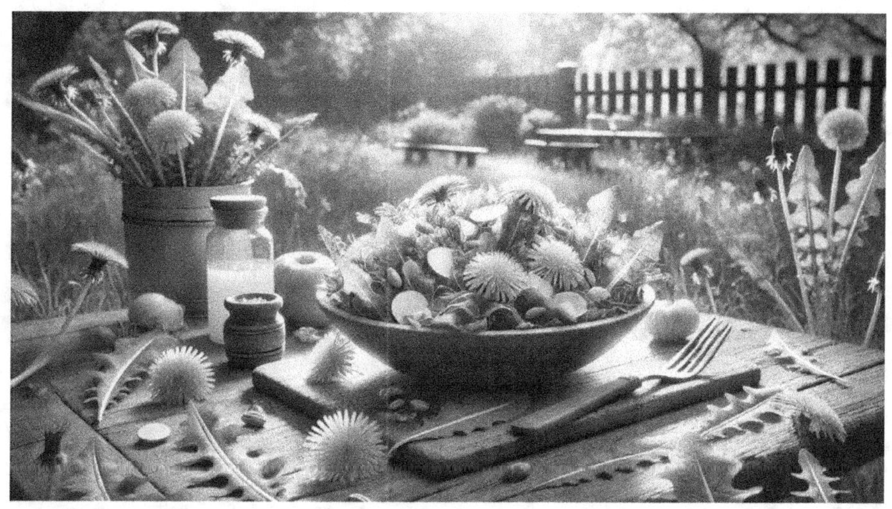

Although dandelions are not ideal for cooking with most foods, you can make them a part of your diet by preparing salads. Here is a simple dandelion salad.

24 thin slices of pancetta

12 mission figs, halved horizontally

6 ounces of chopped dandelion greens, discard the stems

Virgin olive oil for drizzling

1 teaspoon of salt and freshly ground pepper

1 ounce Parmigiano - Reggiano cheese.

Balsamic vinegar

1. Wrap a slice of pancetta around the fig halves and secure with a toothpick.

2. Grill the figs over medium heat until the pancetta is crisp.

3. Transfer the figs to the work surface, remove toothpicks and discard.

4. In a bowl, spread the dandelion leaves, drizzle them with olive oil, and toss.

5. Season your dandelions with salt and pepper.

6. Now arrange the greens on your grill grates and cook on low heat until charred.

7. Transfer the greens to your plate and top with fig halves.

8. Use a vegetable peeler to shave the cheese over your salad and drizzle olive oil and balsamic vinegar and serve.

## LAVENDER RECIPES

Lavender is one of the most popular herbs globally. It is loved due to its sweet scent and can also offer several health benefits. Some of the conditions that can be treated with lavender include anxiety, insomnia, depression, and restlessness, among other conditions.

## LAVENDER TEA

Lavender tea is easy to prepare and can be used to treat most of the above conditions. It is mostly used to treat insomnia and stress. After a long stressful day, prepare a cup of lavender tea to relax your nerves. Here is a simple lavender tea recipe.

4 tablespoons of culinary lavender buds

8 cups of boiling water

1. Place your lavender buds in a pot and pour boiling water over them.

2. Let the lavender steep in hot water for about 10 minutes.

3. Pour your tea through a strainer in a cup and add honey or sugar for sweetening.

Note: You can store any leftover tea in the fridge for about 3 days and warm when you are ready to use it.

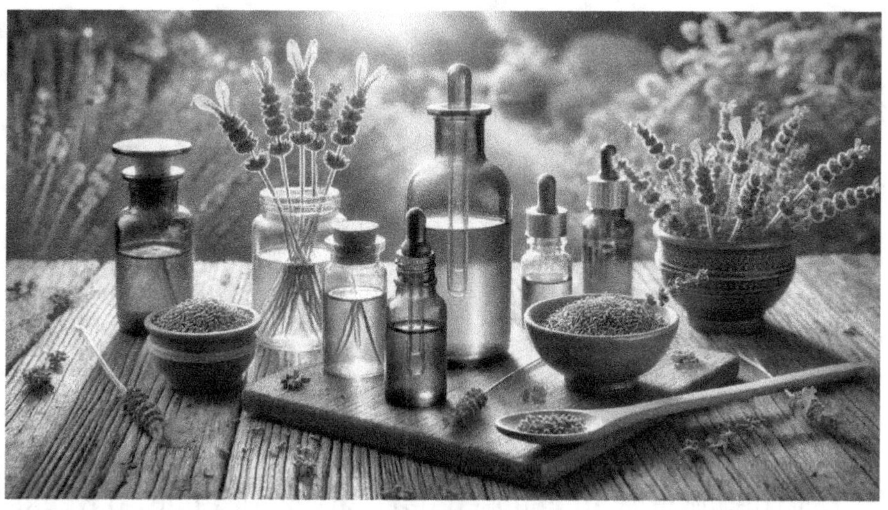

For lavender tincture, you may either use fresh or dried herbs. Here is the recipe for a tincture made with fresh lavender leaves.

1 cup of freshly chopped lavender flowers

Clear vodka, 80 to 100 proof

A clean glass jar with a tight-fitting lid

Fine filter material such as cheesecloth

1. Chop the herbs to increase the surface area to allow them to release essential oils.

2. Fill the jar to the 3/4 mark with the freshly chopped herbs and pack tightly.

3. Pour your vodka over the herbs and cover them completely. However, you should ensure that the herbs move around when slightly agitated.

4. Let the jar stay in a closed dark place for about 6 weeks with occasional shaking throughout the incubation period.

5. After six weeks, strain your herbs into a separate clean jar. Squeeze hard to ensure that you get out as much tincture as possible.

6. Let the tincture settle in the jar for about 4 hours then filter with filter paper.

Store your tincture in a colored glass bottle in a dark place.

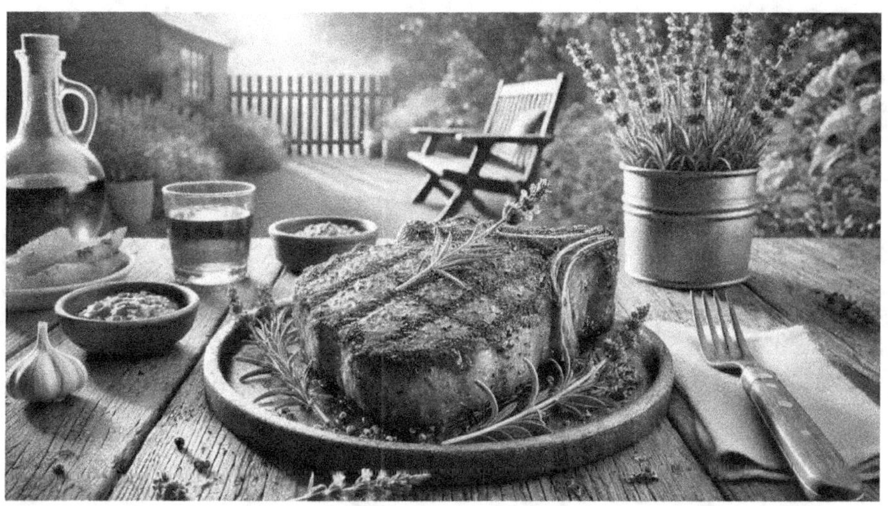

For those who do not enjoy tea or tinctures, you may make lavender part of your daily diet by grilling some steak with the herb. Here is a simple recipe of lavender marinated ribeye steak.

1 tablespoon of dried lavender

1 teaspoon of kosher salt

2/3 cup of champagne vinegar

2/3 cup of extra virgin oil

1/2 teaspoon of chopped fresh thyme

1 teaspoon freshly ground black pepper

2 (1-inch thick) bone-in ribeye steaks

This recipe is divided into 2 sections. We will start by preparing the marinade then grill the steak.

Make the marinade:

1. In a small bowl, crush lavender together with a pinch of salt and add it to the vinegar.

2. Let the lavender steep in the vinegar for about 4 hours. This marinade can be kept in the fridge for at least 5 weeks without going bad.

3. When your marinade is ready, whisk the vinegar with thyme, olive oil, 1/2 teaspoon of salt, and 1/4 teaspoon of pepper.

Marinate the steak:

1. Once you have prepared the marinade, divide it into two. Reserve one half for basting and use the rest to marinate a rib-eye steak. Let your steak stay soaked in the marinade for at least 30 minutes at room temperature or 8 hours in the refrigerator.

2. If you refrigerate your marinade, let the steak come to room temperature before you start preparing.

3. Pat the meat dry and season with salt and pepper before you start grilling.

4. If you are using a charcoal grill, light a chimney starter full of charcoal and bank the coals against one side of the grill. If you are using the gas grill, start with all the burners on medium-high and turn off 1 or more of the burners.

5. Grill your steak at the hottest section of the grill, rotating them occasionally to create a crust. When one

side is well browned, approximately 2 to 4 minutes, turn
the steak and sear the other side.

6. After 4 minutes of grilling both sides of the steak, move
to the cooler part of the grill. Baste the steak occasionally
with the reserved marinade as you desire. Grill on low
heat for about 8 to 12 minutes or until you attain your
desired doneness.

# GINGER RECIPES

Ginger is a popular herb in most homes and is loved due
to its culinary uses. Ginger tea is common in most
cultures and is often used to treat colds. Besides colds,
ginger can also be used medicinally to treat nausea,
arthritis, migraines, and hypertension. Ginger tea is the
best choice for those who wish to treat colds and nausea.
Here are a few recipes for ingesting ginger, including via
a tea and tincture.

Ginger tea is a very important part of herbal medicine. Thankfully, ginger tea can be prepared in just a few steps.

1-inch chunk of freshly sliced ginger rhizome, cut into 1/4-inch slices

1 cup of water

1 piece of cinnamon stick for flavoring

1 thin round of lemon or orange

1 teaspoon of honey or maple syrup

1. Combine the ginger slices with water in a small saucepan and heat over medium-high heat.

2. If you will be adding the cinnamon stick for flavoring to the water immediately when it starts to simmer.

3. Bring the mixture to a boil and reduce the heat to low, allowing the mixture to simmer for about 5 minutes.

4. Remove the saucepan from heat and carefully pour the mixture through a strainer into a heat-safe cup.

Serve your tea in a mug with a lemon slice or drizzle with honey.

## GINGER TINCTURE

This ginger tincture is the best option for those who do not prefer drinking tea. You can prepare your tincture to treat migraines and arthritis. Here is the recipe.

Fresh ginger root, sliced into 1/4 inch slices

1 bottle of 80 proof vodka, about 300ml (about 1 ½ cups)

1. Fill a glass jar to the 3/4 mark with the sliced ginger.

2. Pour the vodka on top of the roots to fill up the jar.

3. Place the lid on the jar and tighten it well and store it in a cool dark place for about 4 weeks.

4. Shake your tincture periodically to allow the ginger to infuse into the vodka completely.

5. After 4 weeks, strain the tincture through a fine sieve or cheesecloth and store in a cool dark place until time to use.

Dosing notes: Since the tincture is much stronger than the tea, you should take it in small amounts. For adults, the recommended dosage is three teaspoons taken three times per day. For children, the recommended dosage is two teaspoons taken twice per day. The tincture is the best option for treating migraines.

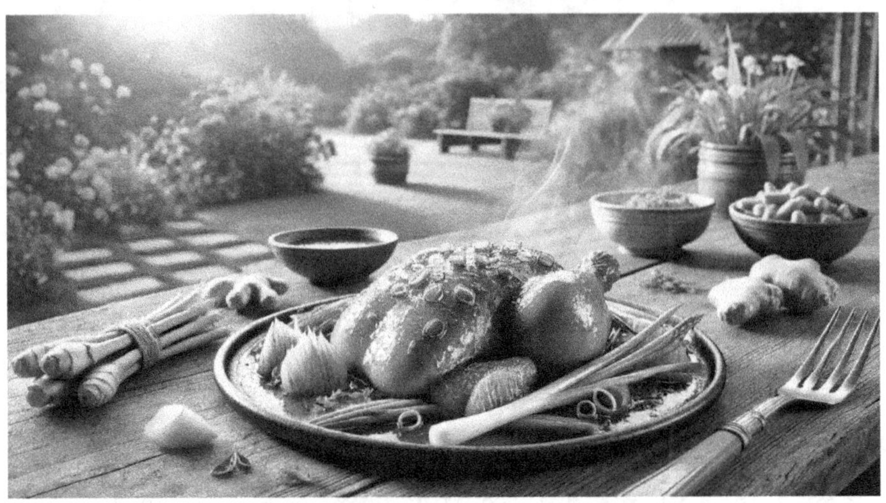

Ginger tea and tincture are mostly prepared to treat a specific condition when it occurs. For most people, ginger tea is only prepared to treat colds. However, ginger has many nutritional and health benefits that you should use on a daily basis. To make ginger part of your daily diet, you should find ways of cooking with ginger. Here is an example of a dish cooked with ginger.

2 lbs. of boneless skinless chicken thighs

1 thumb-size piece of fresh ginger root, peeled and chopped

4 chopped garlic cloves

1 teaspoon of chili powder

½ oz. pack of fresh coriander, chopped

The juice of 1 lime

2 tablespoons of sunflower oil

2 medium-sized onions

1 tablespoon of ground turmeric

1 ½ cups of coconut milk

1 fresh red chili, sliced and deseeded

1 chicken stock cube

1. Cut the chicken thighs into 2 or 3 large chunks and put in a bowl with the ginger, garlic, chili powder, half the coriander, 1 tablespoon, and lime juice. Leave them in the fridge to marinate for about 5 to 12 hours.

2. Peel the onions and finely chopped in a food processor.

3. Heat the remaining oil in a large skillet and add the onions and fry for about 6 minutes or until soft.

4. Add the turmeric, stir, and cook for about 1 more minute

5. Tip in the marinated chicken with the marinade and cook over high heat for about 20 minutes or until the chicken changes color.

6. Pour in the coconut milk, chili, and stock, and cover for about 10 minutes or until the chicken is tender.

7. Add the remaining coriander and stir well. Serve your ginger chicken with rice, a bowl of mango chutney, or bread.

# GARLIC RECIPES

Garlic is a popular spice due to its mouthwatering smell and the ability to make food tasty. Although garlic is a popular herb in most homes, most people do not know how to use it for the medicinal benefits it does offer. Garlic can treat asthma, heart disease, colds, and can boost the immune system.

## GARLIC TEA

Garlic tea is not one of the best teas you will come across. It has a foul smell and a bad test, but it is very beneficial health-wise. If you want to treat colds or any of the conditions mentioned above, here's a recipe for garlic tea.

3 cups of water

3 cloves of garlic- cut in half each.

1/2 cup of honey

1/2 cup of fresh lemon juice

1. In a medium-sized saucepan, combine the cloves of garlic and water and bring to a boil.

2. Once it comes to a boil, turn off the heat and add the 1/2 cup of honey and 1/2 cup of fresh lemon juice.

3. Strain the tea to your cup, and discard the cloves.

Serve the tea while hot and refrigerate the excess for future use.

## GARLIC TINCTURE

Just like all the other herbs, garlic tinctures are the best option for those who do not enjoy teas. Here is the recipe for preparing garlic tinctures.

1 cup of garlic cloves

2 cups of 80 proof vodka

1. Chop the cup of garlic cloves into fine slices and add to a Mason jar.

2. Add 2 cups of vodka to the jar and tighten the lid.

3. Label the jar with the contents and date.

4. Keep the jar in a cool dark place and shake 2 to 3 times every week for 3 weeks.

5. Using a muslin cloth, filter the tincture after 3 weeks and store it in a dark bottle.

You may take the tincture directly, or you may use it in food.

Dosage notes: The dosage for the tincture is about 5 drops once per day for adults. However, children should be given lower doses, such as 2 drops. Do not administer garlic tincture to children under the age of 5 without consulting a doctor.

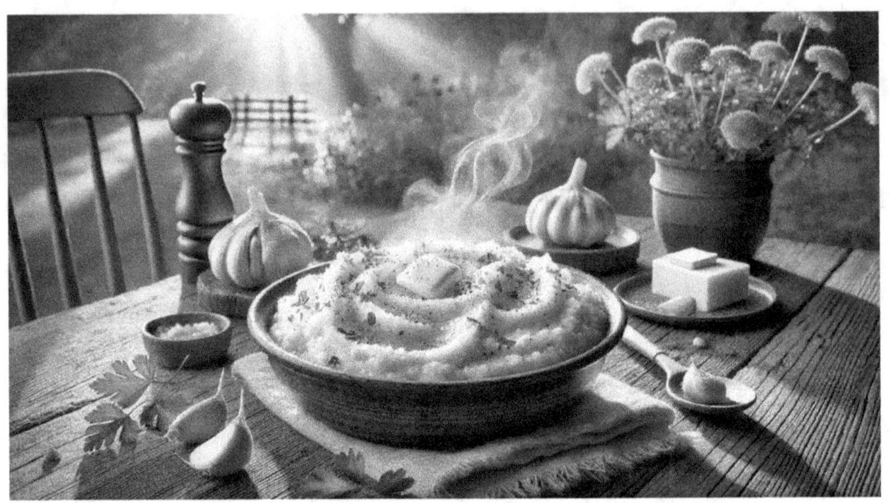

The other option for those who do not enjoy garlic tea or tincture is cooking with garlic. The best part is that garlic can be used to cook almost all types of foods. Here is the recipe for garlic mashed potatoes.

2 lbs. of potatoes, peeled and quartered

Butter for frying

1 garlic clove finely chopped

½ cup heavy cream

2 tablespoons dried bread crumbs

¼ cup of gruyere cheese, grated

2 thyme sprigs, strip the leaves

1. Cook your potatoes in a large skillet for about 10 to 15 minutes or until soft.

2. Drain your potatoes well and set them aside.

3. Place the pan back on the heat, melt the butter, and use it for cooking the garlic for about 1 minute.

4. Stir in the cream and heat through for about 3 minutes.

5. Now return the potatoes into the cooked garlic and mash until smooth.

6. Once your potatoes are smoothly mashed, heat your oven to about 200 degrees F.

7. Spoon the potatoes onto a baking sheet and sprinkle the top with breadcrumbs, cheese, and thyme.

8. Once ready, you may cook immediately in the oven, or you may refrigerate overnight before baking. (This makes a great make-ahead dish!)

9. Once ready for baking, bake in the oven for 15 minutes for those who bake immediately after mashing. If you bake after refrigeration, you have to cook for about 1 hour and 10 minutes.

# VALERIAN RECIPES

Valerian is not one of the most popular herbs on this list, but it offers plenty of benefits. This herb can be used to prepare herbal tea and other foods. Some of the benefits of valerian include reducing heavy menstrual flow, stopping bleeding, reducing menstrual pain, and treatment of low blood pressure.

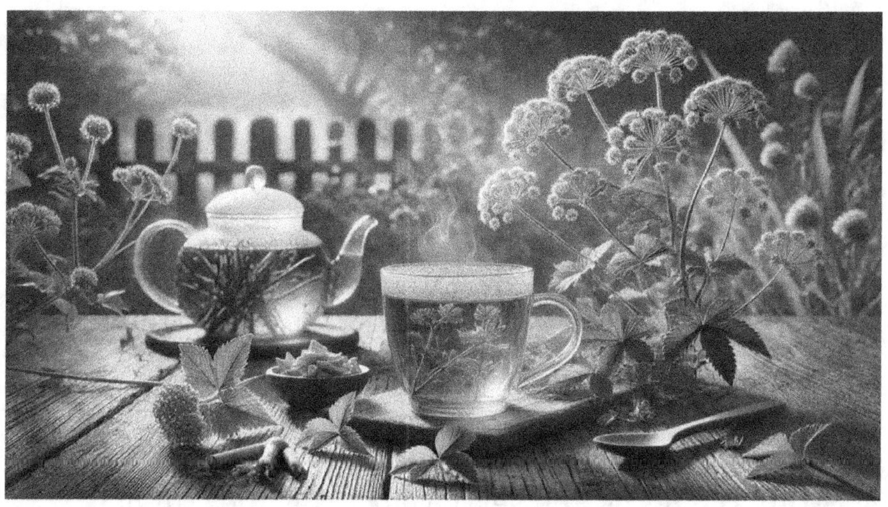

Since valerian is a bitter herb, it is mixed with other herbs to prepare medicinal tea that is palatable. Here is a recipe for the healthy valerian tea.

1 teaspoon of lemon balm

4 teaspoons of licorice root

1 quart of water

2 teaspoons of valerian leaves

1. Place the licorice roots in a small saucepan with 1 quart of cold water.

2. Simmer the licorice roots over low heat for about 15minutes.

3. Remove the licorice from the heat and add the valerian leaves and lemon balm to the saucepan and let them steep for about 45 minutes.

4. Strain the herbs and serve your tea while still hot.

You may add sugar or honey to taste.

## VALERIAN TINCTURE

A valerian tincture is easy to prepare and can treat most of the conditions mentioned above. Here is the recipe.

4 tablespoons of passionflower, dried

4 tablespoons of valerian root, dried

500ml (about 2 cups) of 100 proof vodka

1. Add the dried herbs to a sterilized glass jar to about 3/4 mark. Fill up the glass jar with vodka and label it with the date and the contents of the bottle.

2. Fasten the lid on the glass jar and store your tincture in a cool dark place.

3. Let the tincture infuse for about 6 weeks with occasional shaking.

4. After 6 weeks of infusion, decant the tincture into a clean glass jar.

5. Now filter the tincture through a fine sieve or cheesecloth.

Store your tincture in a dark bottle for use for up to 3 years.

Finally, you may choose to use valerian roots to prepare your daily meals. Many meals can be prepared with valerian. A good example is poached salmon. Here is the recipe.

7 ounces of salmon

3 sprigs of green onions (scallions)

Juice of half a lime

1 tablespoon of black peppercorns

1 cup of water

1 ounce of pine nuts

6 ounces of valerian

4 radishes, thinly sliced

1 tablespoon of olive oil

1 tablespoon of vinegar

1. Heat your skillet over medium heat and place your salmon in the skillet skin down.

2. Add the sprig, onions, lime juice, and black peppercorns.

3. Add the water and bring the dish to a boil. Once the dish boils, reduce the heat and let it simmer for about 4 minutes.

4. Flip the salmon on the other side and continue cooking for about 5 minutes.

5. In a separate skillet, toss the pine nuts for about 1 minute.

6. Now place your valerian into a bowl and add the radish slices and the toasted pine nuts.

7. Using a knife, peel off the skin of the salmon and use your hands to break small threads off the salmon.

8. Add the threads of salmon on top of your salad and season the salad with olive oil, vinegar, and salt.

## PRESERVATION AND STORAGE

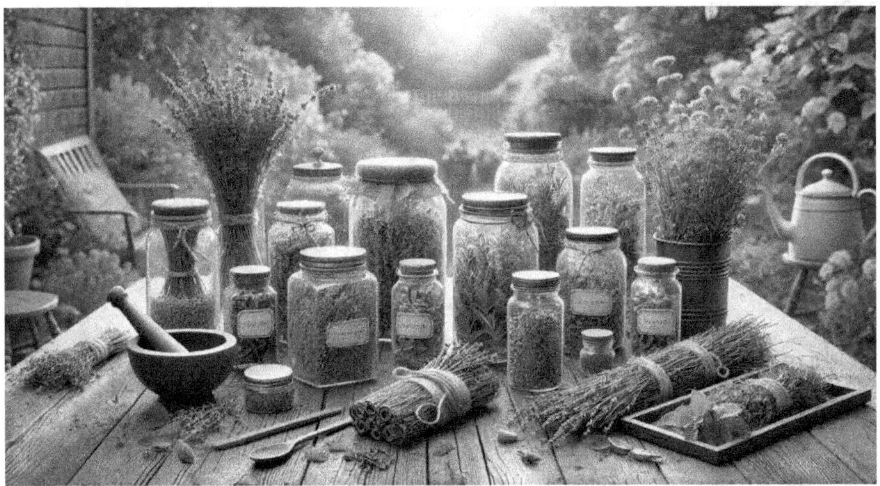

After harvesting your herbs and preparing several recipes, you have to store them in the right way. There are many ways of preserving herbs for future use. One of the ways is by preparing herbal tinctures. As we have seen, most of the tinctures can be used for a period of 1 to

3 years, while others can last up to 6 years without going bad. However, you might also want to preserve the herbs in their natural state. Here are some ways you may follow in preserving herbs in their natural state.

## AIR DRYING

Drying herbs is the easiest way of preservation. The drying process should be slow so that the nutritional components of the herb are not damaged. To air-dry the herbs, collect the herbs (stalks or leaves), and hang them in a warm room. The ideal place for air drying herbs is the kitchen. In the kitchen, you can hang the herbs in the air so that they can dry slowly in the warm environment. Air drying should take about 3 weeks for the herbs to completely dry. After air drying, store your herbs in a Mason jar in a cool, dry place for as long as you wish.

## MICROWAVE DRYING

The alternative to air drying is microwave drying. Microwave drying is helpful for those who live in moist and damp regions. You may either use a microwave or a dehydrator. To dry your herbs in the microwave, just place the leaves or sprigs onto a paper towel and cover with another layer of paper towel. Place them into the microwave and microwave on high for about 2 to 3 minutes. Check the herbs every 30 seconds and rearrange them accordingly to ensure that they dry on all sides. Let the herbs cool for about 30 minutes before storing in an airtight Mason jar in a cool dark place. Just like air-dried herbs, microwaved herbs can last for as long as you wish.

## FREEZING HERBS

Besides drying herbs, you could also freeze them. Most fleshy herbs such as aloe vera, basil, parsley, and cilantro can be frozen and stored for a very long time. To freeze your herbs, blanch them in boiling water for several seconds before placing them into a bowl of ice-cold water. Remove from the ice water, pat all the sides with dish towels and pack them into freezer bags. Place the herbs in the freezer for a lifespan of up to 2 years. When you want to use the herbs, remove from the freezer, and give them about 30 minutes before you use them.

The other option when it comes to the storage of herbs is by using ice cubes. You can store your herbs in ice cube trays by mixing the herbs with water. Just add chopped herbs to your ice cube tray so that each tray is half full. Top up the tray with water and freeze. Let your herbs stay frozen for as long as you wish. When you are ready to use the herbs, remove the ice cube tray from the freezer and let the ice cubes melt in a jar. Strain out the herbs and use them accordingly.

## Frozen Blends

Besides freezing the herbs, you may also freeze the blended version of the herbs. For instance, instead of placing the herbs into the ice tray, you may blend the herbs with oil and pour them into ice cube trays. To preserve space for your ice cubes, pop the blend out once they dry and store in freezer bags.

The other way of storing herbs is by preparing butter or tinctures. To store your herbs in butter, leave a part of butter at room temperature to soften. Once soft, chop your favorite herb leaves and mash them into the butter. Keep the butter at room temperature for use up to 2 days. Refrigerate for use up to a week and freeze for use up to six months.

Besides the preparation of herbal butter, you can also preserve your herbs by preparing tinctures. We have looked at the process of preparing all the tinctures.

## VINEGAR AND OILS

Herbs that are stored in butter and oil can exclude oxygen and increase the risk of botulism. To avoid the risk, you may store your herbs in vinegar. As we have already seen, vinegar is an active ingredient that can be used to prepare tinctures. However, you can also use vinegar to preserve herbs without necessarily having to prepare tinctures. To preserve your herbs, soak your finely

shredded herbs in vinegar and mix with some cooking oil
if you choose to prepare salad dressing. This option just
allows you to lock in summer freshness for about 1 year.
There are other methods of preserving herbs, such as
blanching, preserving in sugar, and herbal wines.

# CHAPTER 5: PRECAUTIONS WHEN USING HERBAL MEDICINE

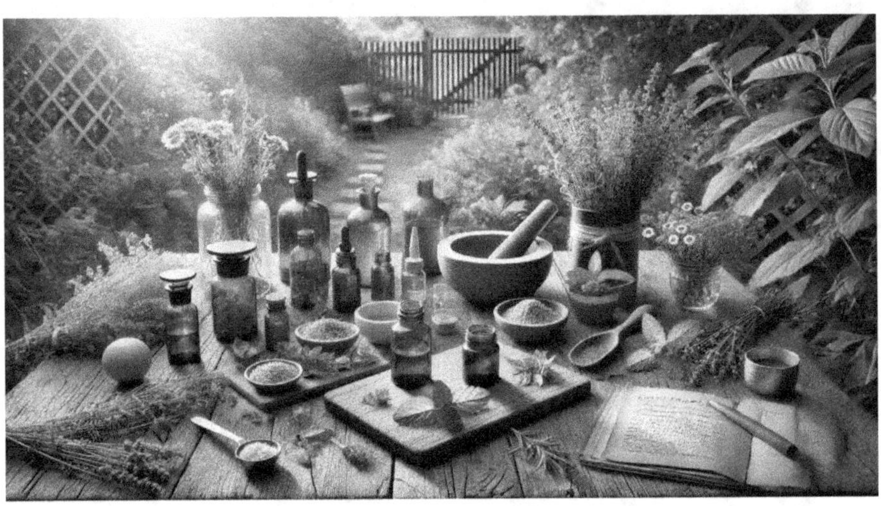

While herbal medicine is considered safer than pharmaceutical drugs, some herbs have side effects that may vary from person to person. You should be cautious when planting and using herbs. Some herbal products are too strong and may cause side effects in some people. In this chapter, we will be looking at ways to use herbal drugs without endangering your life. There are also cautions to be taken when preparing herbal consumables such as tea and tinctures.

# Risks Involved in Using Herbs as Medicine

Using herbal plants presents some risks to the users. Some of the risks you will have to deal with include:

## Inaccurate Dosage

One of the risks involved in using herbal medicine is dosages. For some herbs, using in large amounts presents serious side effects. Unfortunately, there is no accurate way of dosage. For instance, you are required to take just 2 droppers of ginger tincture per day. However, 2 droppers of ginger may contain different quantities of the medicinal compounds. If one person uses too much alcohol in preparing the tincture, the quality of the tincture might be too strong, and taking 2 droppers might lead to overdosing. In general, doses for most herbs are estimations. Such estimations can get out of hand and lead to some side effects.

The other risk involved in using herbal medicine is skipping doses. Skipping a dose can occur if you're away from home and did not bring along your herbs. Herbs are not easily available in all regions. This means that you have to carry your herbs everywhere you go. If you cannot carry your herbs, prepare portable herbal eatables such as tinctures to help you always carry your herbs with you.

Once a person gets used to a certain herb, they may experience side effects if the daily dosage is missed. For instance, feverfew is used to treat fevers and migraines. If you get used to taking feverfew tea every morning, you should not miss it. Once you skip the dosage, you are likely to experience a headache throughout the day. To avoid such risks, make sure you have portable herbs at all times. In case you find yourself in a distant place without your herbs, shop for them in local stores to ensure that you do not skip the dosage.

The other risk of using herbs is that they may have unknown side effects. As we have mentioned, it was not until the early 21st century that modern scientists started researching herbal medicine. Initially, most people had assumed that herbal plants do not have any value. In my years of research, I have realized that we know very little about most herbal plants. Some herbs we use are only taken due to their perceived health benefits. Some of the benefits of other herbs are not known.

At the same time, some serious side effects of the herbs are not known. The research data available today do not give a conclusive analysis of most herbs. Therefore, people who suffer from certain conditions may react differently to certain herbs. Herbal medicine might cause allergic reactions that are not known. Some herbs may also affect people who use certain drugs without knowing.

The other risk of dealing with herbs without having a full scientific understanding of their functions is that you may combine harmful herbs. While some drugs work well independently, they are harmful when combined with others. The same case applies to herbal medicine. There are some herbs that offer conflicting effects on the body. If you use two herbs with conflicting effects on the body, chances are that you may experience some side effects.

## Herbs with Pharmaceutical Medicine

The other risk involved in using herbal medicine is a case where you end up combining harmful herbs with pharmaceutical drugs. For instance, it is not recommended to use anticoagulants with heart disease medicine. If you are on heart disease medication, you should only use herbs that stimulate the blood under the guidance of a doctor. If you are using any drugs, you should get permission from your doctors before you make any decisions about using herbal drugs.

There are no specific guidelines to follow when prescribing herbal drugs. When it comes to herbal medicine, there are two recommended ways of ingestion: food-based consumption and drug-based consumption. Since taking too much of any drug can be harmful, herbal drugs are best taken in food. However, herbs can also be taken directly as drugs. You may either take the tinctures or chew the herbs directly. These ways of consumption of herbal products make it difficult to attain the right dosage. To ensure that you get the right dosage, I usually recommend sticking to diet based herbal consumption.

## DIET BASED DOSAGE

For an herbal-based diet, the dosage is very simple. Just follow the recipe, and you will have no problem. I recommend herbal-based diets because they are more effective than taking drugs. If you use herbs as part of your lifestyle, they help prevent many diseases and cause fewer side effects. The beauty of diet based herbal medicine is that you can never overdose. When herbs are a part of your diet, they will be used in limited amounts.

In most cases, we only use one leaf or a few leaves of herbs to ensure that they do not interfere with the taste of the food. However, if you have to take the herb as a drug directly, you have to take care not to overdose. For all those who are thinking about introducing herbs to their life, I will recommend starting slowly. Start with the lowest dosage possible used in foods. As you advance, monitor the effects of the herbs on your body and increase the dosage to the level that works.

## DOSAGE OF HERBAL TINCTURE

Tinctures and other ingestible are the ideal choices for all people who do not prefer taking herbs in foods. Tinctures present a more concentrated version of any herb and are likely to provide fast results. The only downside of using herbal tinctures is that they can easily be overdosed and cause side effects. Furthermore, the dosage that works for one person might not work for another. Therefore, every person must find a dosage that works for them.

Just like it is the case with diet based herbal consumption, taking tinctures and other herbal drugs requires a slow approach. Do not just start by taking the recommended dosage if you're a beginner. Start slow and monitor your progress as you move on. If you are using the herbs to treat chronic pain such as arthritis, you should take small amounts and monitor the effects. If you feel that the small amount works for your case, do not increase the dosage. For tincture, I recommend starting at 2 to 3 droppers of the herb. If they do not have a serious effect on your condition, increase the dosage day after day until you feel the effect. However, do not worry so much about herbal teas. You can consume the herbal tea at any time as long you stick to the provided recipes when brewing your tea.

## COMBINING HERBAL MEDICINE WITH MODERN MEDICINE

There is a misconception that herbal medicine is natural and does not have any effect when consumed with pharmaceutical drugs. As it turns out, most herbs are harmful when combined with some medicine. Some herbal drugs can react with modern drugs and present a totally different result from the anticipated results.

One way that herbal drugs affect pharmaceutical drugs is that they may reduce or increase the rate of metabolism. When pharmaceutical drugs are prepared, they are designed to offer treatment within a given period of time. If you affect the expected absorption time of the drug, chances are that it may not be effective. To ensure that your drugs are not affected in terms of metabolism, avoid all herbs that increase blood flow or detoxify the body while on medication. Such herbs may affect metabolism and make the drugs ineffective.

Besides affecting the rate of metabolism, herbal drugs may also reduce the effectiveness of a drug. If a drug is absorbed much faster than it is recommended, it will turn out to be less effective. At the same time, if a drug is absorbed much slower than recommended, it will not provide the anticipated results. Just like pharmaceutical drugs, herbal medicine can alter the normal functioning of the body too. If the body functions are altered, there are high chances that the drug will not be effective in treating the condition it was meant to treat.

For instance, researchers have established that a common herb, St John's Wort, can affect the effectiveness of some drugs. The herb is used as an antidepressant and is often prescribed over the counter. However, when taken with drugs that require a stimulated system, it reduces their effectiveness. St John's Wort has been confirmed to reduce the effectiveness of warfarin, statins, antihistamines, birth control, and HIV medication. When such drugs are taken simultaneously with St John's Wort, they are not absorbed in the recommended rate and are less effective.

All herbal drugs are discouraged for individuals who are on heart disease medication. Several studies have revealed that heart disease medicine does not work well with green teas and herbs. For instance, patients who suffer from heart problems and on warfarin or statins should not use herbal drugs. If such patients use herbs such as ginger, cayenne, or any of the stimulating herbs, they risk suffering from heart attacks.

Besides those who suffer from her attacks, it's also important to avoid using herbal medicine completely if you are on drugs for any chronic condition. If you suffer from diabetes, heart disease, HIV, or any condition that requires continued medication, you should never use herbal products. If you have to use herbs in your condition, make sure you consult your doctor. Some herbs may inhibit the functions of your regular drugs and lead to further complications.

Most importantly, special groups of people such as kids below the age of 5, pregnant mothers, and lactating mothers should never use herbal medicine without consulting the doctor. Most kids are weak and at the risk of sickness. If you start using substances that may have side effects on your child, it will not take long before your child falls sick. Avoid complications by staying away from herbal medicine unless recommended by your doctor.

## IS HERBAL MEDICINE ALWAYS SAFE SINCE IT IS NATURAL?

The assumption that herbal medicine is always safe because it is natural is a myth. In reality, all drugs have side effects. However, herbal medicines do have fewer side effects as compared to pharmaceutical ones. People who use herbal medicine are less likely to encounter far-reaching side effects. With that said, always ensure that you take the recommended dose of all herbal drugs and monitor your body to see if the drug causes any side effects.

## HOW EFFECTIVE ARE HERBAL ANTIMICROBIALS?

The other myth about herbal medicine is that they are not effective antimicrobials. Herbal medicine works very well in preventing the spread of microorganisms. On our list of herbs, you can use garlic or oregano as the best antimicrobial drugs.

## WHAT ARE THE DISADVANTAGES OF HERBAL MEDICINES?

Just like pharmaceutical medicines, herbal drugs also have disadvantages. Some of the disadvantages include improper dosage, lack of sufficient scientific data, unknown side effects, among others. When using herbal medicine, you should keep in mind that most of the drugs are not well known in terms of scientific research. They may have hidden side effects and benefits.

## IS IT POSSIBLE TO ESTIMATE THE QUANTITY OF AN HERB OR HERBAL EXTRACT ADDED IN AN HERBAL PRODUCT?

Yes, it is possible to estimate the quantity of herbal extract added to a product. If you are using herbal supplements, have a look at the ingredients that the supplement contains. If the product is genuine, there should be a clear label of the amount of herbal extract used. If you are the one preparing the product, let's say you are brewing herbal tea, you can also estimate the quantity of herbal extract in your tea. To avoid a situation where you brew tea but do not know how much herbal extract the tea contains, use soluble herbal extracts such as tinctures to prepare the tea. You will be in a position to quantify exactly how much herbs you have used.

## DO ALCOHOLIC PREPARATIONS INTERACT WITH PLASTIC CONTAINERS AND BECOME TOXIC?

Yes. As you can see from all our recipes above, we recommend preparing your tinctures in a glass bottle. We also recommend storing the final product in a glass bottle. In most cases, plastic may react with the alcohol used in preparing tinctures and leak toxic substances into your tincture. If you must use plastic in preparing herbal products, choose food-grade plastic. Even with that said, glass bottles are ideal for many reasons. With the glasses, you can see inside the bottle to determine the progress of the infusion. Even though looking through a colored glass might be a challenge, it is much simpler than looking through a colored plastic bottle.

# CONCLUSION

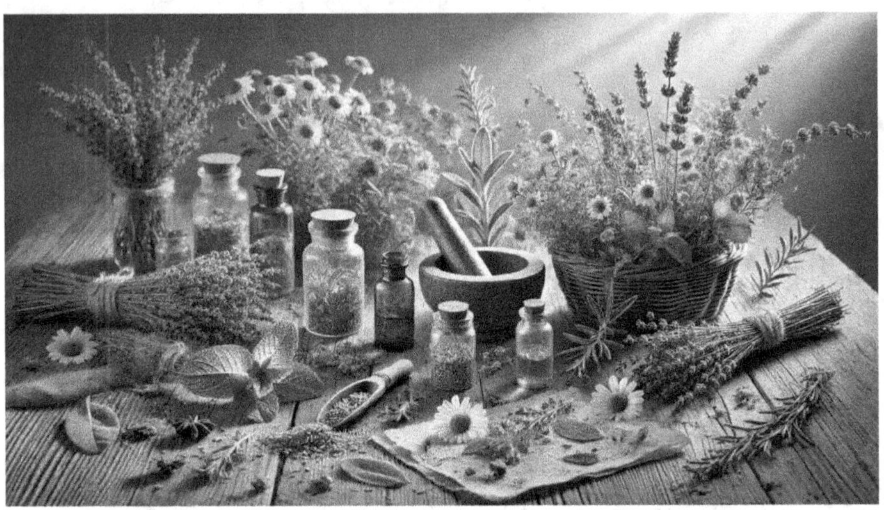

Congratulations on reading this book to the end. At this point, you have sharpened your skills in regard to planting, caring, and harvesting herbal plants. You have also advanced your knowledge in regard to using herbal products and preparing herbal ingestible. This book is prepared to help those who have an interest in living a healthy life by using herbal medicine. The book seeks to answer questions regarding the authenticity of herbal drugs and the possibility of using herbal drugs to treat common ailments.

Having gone through the whole book to the end, I am confident that you have acquired skills that will help you plant, maintain, and use herbs. The book mainly covers two key areas: planting and caring for herbs and the application of herbal medicine. In the book, we have looked at all the steps you should take before and during herbal farming. We have looked at the beneficial herbs you can plant, when, and where to plant them. We have outlined the ways to care for your herbal crops, how to maintain them in harsh seasons, and how to harvest. The book gives you a detailed outlook on how to ensure that your herbs thrive. It indicates the right time to plant your herbs so that they can thrive and also indicates the ideal conditions under which specific herbs thrive.

In the second section of the book, we mainly focus on harvesting, storage, and preparation of herbal products. Each of the herbs listed in this book has an ideal way of harvesting, storage, and preparation. We have looked at over 25 recipes, including herbal teas, herbal tinctures, and herbal dishes. All these recipes give you ways of consuming herbs. We have looked at the dosages and the way to ensure that you do not take more herbal products than recommended. At the end of the book, we have looked at the precautions you must take when using herbal products. Although most herbs are harmless, they may have some side effects on specific groups of people. We have highlighted the groups of people who should never use herbal medicine and when they are allowed to use herbs.

If you are interested in herbal medicine in any way, this book is ideal for you. It separates the myths from the facts, provides detailed ways of planting and caring for herbs, and shows you the best ways to use your herbs. You should not look anywhere else if you wish to find out more about backyard herbal gardens and home remedies for all conditions.

Thank you for taking the time to read, and good luck in all your ventures.

If this book has been beneficial to you in any way, would you please consider leaving a review online where you purchased the book? Online reviews really help me in reaching more readers, and I can gain valuable feedback. Thank you in advance!

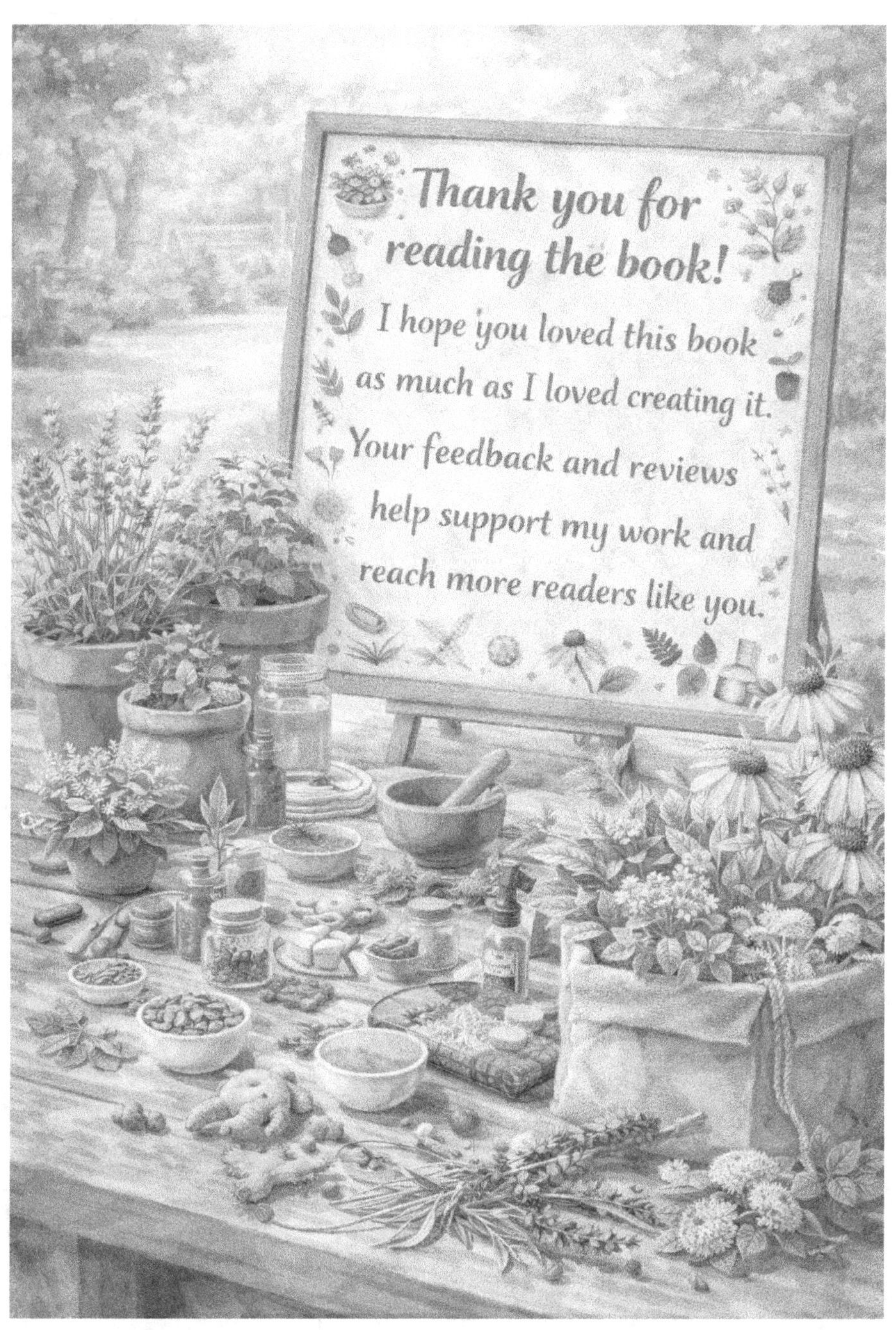

Thank you for reading the book!
I hope you loved this book as much as I loved creating it.
Your feedback and reviews help support my work and reach more readers like you.